The
REFLEXOLOGY
PARTNERSHIP

Suzanne Adamson was a registered nurse and health visitor before qualifying as a Reflex Zone Therapist. She has been practising with and learning from her clients for the last ten years. She is a part-time health visitor for the Camden and Islington Community Health Services NHS Trust and development officer/therapist for the charity SCOPE, which provides alternative therapies for people with disabilities.

Eilish Harris, a qualified nurse, was drawn to reflexology in 1982 while seeking treatment for a frozen shoulder. For the last twelve years she has studied reflexology and in particular the relationship between the reflexologist and client. She has a grown-up son and daughter.

The REFLEXOLOGY PARTNERSHIP

A HEALING BOND

SUZANNE ADAMSON & EILISH HARRIS

WITH SHARRON KERR

Illustrations by Sally Maltby

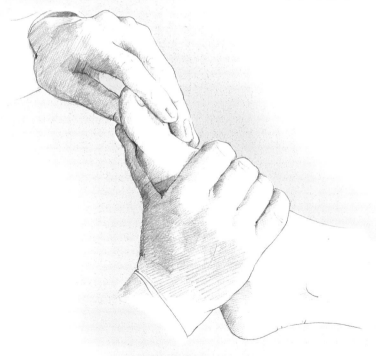

KYLE CATHIE LIMITED

First published in Great Britain by
Kyle Cathie Limited
20 Vauxhall Bridge Road
London SW1V 2SA

ISBN 1 85626 149 2

Suzanne Adamson, Eilish Harris and Sharron Kerr are hereby identified as the authors of this work in accordance with Section 77 of the Copyright, Designs and Patents Act 1988

A Cataloguing in Publication record for this title is available from the British Library

Designed by Geoff Hayes

Printed and Bound in Great Britain
by The Bath Press

Cover illustration © John Garrett

Dedication

To Suzanne's husband, Tommy, and Eilish's sister, Margaret, who through dying taught us so much about living.

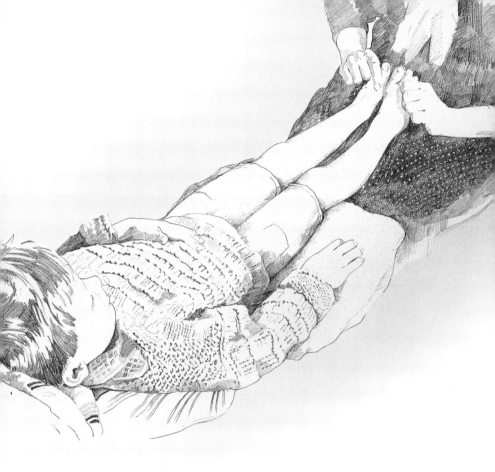

Acknowledgements

It is a great pleasure to acknowledge the help and support we have
received from Christine Issel, whose research into the history of
reflexology has been an invaluable resource for us, Roger Coghill, Jazz
Rasool, Ann Jordan, the Association of Reflexologists, the Danish
Reflexologist's Association and the Chinese Preventive Medicine
Association. This work would not have been possible without the patient
advice and technical help of Sharron Kerr, Sally Maltby, Stephanie Darnill,
Tom Murdoch, Sarah Stacey, Colin McLaren and John Goldman. Finally,
we would like to thank all those people who have been partners in
reflexology, and our family and friends for their understanding and
forebearance during the writing of this book.

CONTENTS

Acknowledgements   6
Introduction   9

Chapter 1
REFLEXOLOGY THEN AND NOW   16

Chapter 2
HOW DOES IT WORK?   26

Chapter 3
TOUCH AND THE REFLEXOLOGY PARTNERSHIP   41

Chapter 4
HOW REFLEXOLOGY CAN HELP YOU   53

Chapter 5
HOW TO FIND YOUR THERAPIST   68

Chapter 6
HOW REFLEXOLOGY CAN HELP YOU HELP YOURSELF   83

Conclusion   92
Useful Addresses   94
Bibliography   95
Index   96

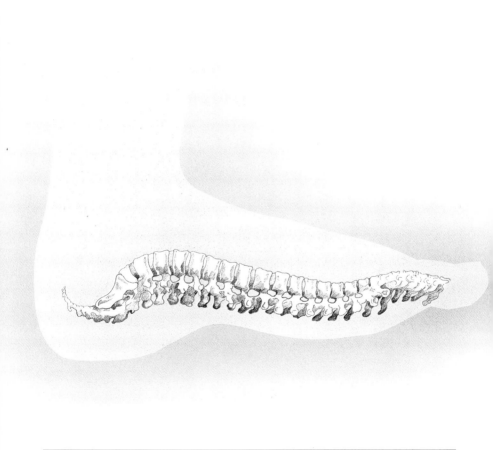

Introduction

Reflexology is an ancient form of foot massage based on the belief that our bodies are reflected in miniature in our feet and that by massaging the different parts of our feet we can affect our state of health and general well-being.

Each one of us is made up of energy vibrating at various frequencies. In other cultures the existence of this energy has long been formally acknowledged and is now being recognized here. There are words for it in both the Chinese and Indian languages. The Chinese term is *qi* and the Indian name is *prana*, and we know it as the life force. The slowest vibration is represented by our physical body and this is a reflection of the subtle energy bodies surrounding us that vibrate at faster frequencies and are not visible. Your subtle energy is the energy that surrounds you as a sheath. Have you ever wondered why if someone is standing behind you, for example, you can suddenly become aware of the person's presence? This is not necessarily brought to your attention by your hearing but you sense the presence through the contact of two subtle energy fields. Or rub your hands together, hold them apart and then slowly bring your palms together, paying attention to any sensations you may experience. Most people are usually aware of a tingling sensation or a feeling of substance as if there is some force between your hands. This is a simple method of experiencing this non-visible energy.

Life force or basic energy is found in everything. It vibrates at different rates or frequencies and its physical manifestation can be seen around us as plants, flowers, animals, people, stones and soil. Human beings have an added dimension in intelligence which gives us the ability to utilize the energy in a way which can enhance life or destroy life.

In all living matter the life force is differentiated to create the different cells which perform separate functions. For instance the cells in the retina of the eye are different from those in the heart. The cells in the retina are specifically adapted to react to light so that an image is formed of the object observed while the heart cell's function is to keep the pump going.

The primary spark comes into physical existence at conception and is nourished and replenished by the food we eat, the air we breathe, our mental activity which includes our thoughts, our friends, our work, how we spend our leisure, what clothes we wear, colours and the environment that we exist and live in.

Higher vibrations that permeate all manifestations are invisible; although they can be difficult to understand they are the organising force that sustains life. Mystics have described its importance and now proved its existence, and are continuously discovering new aspects in Quantum Physics. The heart is the bridge that unites the higher energy with lower physical energy, or heaven and earth.

The acceptance of the basic principle that the body has an intricate network of linking pathways, known as meridians in acupuncture, is common to several traditions of ancient holistic treatment. These treatments are based on the philosophy that a balanced state of this energy is the key to good health.

In reflexology the therapist's intention is to facilitate the balancing of this energy. Through the feet, or hands, reflexologists can help to identify blockages of energy and by massage assist the person to deal with this state of imbalance in the body. Touch is the medium which provides this valuable strategy for health care, relaxation, regeneration and well-being. Often we respond to the pressures of life by automatically taking an 'on-guard' stance, and, as a result, constrict the easy flow of the body's vital energy. Though a certain amount of stress is healthy, when it goes on unabated it can be destructive, thus leading to a state of distress in which dis-ease can develop.

Many people who lead demanding lives have turned to reflexology as a regular practice. We recall a singer, basically healthy but struggling with the debilitating effects of constant travel, getting off the couch and saying, with relief, 'Now I can sing'. Other people who have experienced reflexology often say that they understand their body better, and they recognize how their physical functions affect them socially, mentally and emotionally and vice versa. One man claimed that, after stressful events, reflexology gives him the strength not to give in but to keep on going. 'It bats me back' is the way he describes it.

Our roads to reflexology and understanding the healing bond that can be achieved through this type of massage have been quite different. We are both nurses and mothers with differing back-grounds and life experiences. Perhaps coincidentally, we both have fond and vivid memories of running free and barefoot as children. So from that initial basic awareness of our feet, our journeys to discovering reflexology have been different but they have brought us to the same destination and the same ultimate convictions.

Suzanne spent nine years as a racehorse trainer in Kenya where she became increasingly aware of the importance of touch. She observed how horses, for instance, appreciated the quality of touch and that some people had an innate capacity to interact even with difficult horses. It was as if they were in a state of unconscious attention, totally 'with' the horse. Animals cannot be hoodwinked and they respond to the quality of the touch they are experiencing.

She then moved to Britain where she resumed work as a midwife and later trained as a health visitor. She was troubled by what she saw as the negative effects of medication on elderly people, and children in particular. In 1984 this concern turned her towards complementary therapies and that was when she decided to study reflexology and how to get the most from it.

Now her time is shared between working for the charity SCOPE, which offers complementary therapies to people with physical disablement, and a London NHS Trust as a part-time health visitor, running a baby massage group and introducing complementary therapies. She also runs a small private practice.

For the last twelve years Eilish has been exploring and trying to learn about the therapy and in particular the importance of the relationship between reflexologist and therapee. Therapee is an expressive word which we have decided to use instead of client, patient and customer with all their inherent implications.

Eilish was first drawn to reflexology in 1982 while seeking help for a very painful frozen shoulder. Although receiving excellent orthodox medical treatment she intuitively felt that this was not identifying the underlying cause of her discomfort. She realised that there were other ways of dealing with the pain and immobility and decided to explore them.

She tried reflexology and became very excited by this therapy and the new holistic approach to healing that it offered her. She found it very comforting and after a few weeks the pain in her shoulder subsided and movement in her arm became freer than it had ever been before. The therapy also lifted her emotionally and she felt able to be herself rather than the way other people wanted her to be. As a result of her experience she decided to discover more about the potent effects of touch through reflexology.

She did an introductory course and was very interested. Then after considering what was available she chose a course that offered training to those who had qualifications of a medical background. This short course opened up new areas in connection with health and illness that she had not thought of before and provided a sound base on which to build. Now it has become clear that while the medical model has a prime place in healthcare reflexology is based on a different philosophy and though still in its infancy promises to develop and take its place, especially in the early stages of dis-ease.

Eilish has worked voluntarily in hospitals offering reflexology to people who were seriously ill. At the beginning she was known as the 'foot lady' to many of those she came into contact with. With her growing confidence and beliefs in the benefits of reflexology, to be known as the foot lady is music to her ears.

Through our years of working with people – be it in the hospital setting as nurses or as reflexology practitioners – we have observed and considered the hidden processes involved in healing, the necessary relationship which is a partnership between the therapist and the therapee.

We appreciate the value of orthodox medicine. It is indispensable and life-saving. But we have realised that there is a lot more to ill-health and its treatment than conventional medicine caters for. In particular, it neglects the importance of touch and communication. For example, if someone cannot sleep try rubbing their back; if someone is lonely or depressed talk to them and listen to them, do not just administer pills. Conventional medicine aims to make you better by removing the symptoms of illness. Reflexology can take you beyond being better merely because the symptoms of illness have been removed, beyond the state of functional wellness to a whole new sense of well-being.

In reflexology there is a blurring of the division between practitioner and the person having reflexology – there is no 'sufferer' and 'curer', no 'submissive' role and 'dominant' role. Both sides must respond to the needs and feelings of the other. The reflexology partnership is in essence a relationship between two people who share equally with each other in order to facilitate change. That is why it is so important to find the right reflexologist, the one who suits you.

While discussing our observations and aspirations for the role of reflexology in the future, we do not want to put ourselves up as experts. We want to discuss our understanding of reflexology as it is now. This book is an effort, in the light of our experience, to explore the unfolding aspects of the healing partnership in reflexology. Who knows what the understanding of health will be in five years' time?

This book is aimedspecifically at the person who is considering a course of treatment and who wants to find out more about the subject so they can make the right choices. We also want to communicate our concerns that in trying to achieve recognition in the eyes of orthodox medicine reflexology is being conventionalized and 'medicalized' in order to provide it with acceptability. There are certain things in life for which one must stop needing explanations and be content that they just happen; reflexology makes people feel better just because it does.

Reflexology offers a completely different approach to health and illness, to ease and dis-ease, and thus needs its own identity. You cannot buy and you cannot sell health. Health is a process not a commodity. We believe that reflexology is able to stand alone and be credited for its vital role in modern healthcare.

There is now a groundswell of interest in health and dis-ease and people are becoming more informed, increasingly responsible and taking an active interest in their own health. The market is flooded with books and articles related to various therapies, thus making choices between them confusing. We hope this book gives those considering the therapy a broad picture of reflexology that enables them to decide if it is right for them and also to find a therapist with whom they feel comfortable.

Chapter 1
Reflexology Then and Now

You may be forgiven for thinking that reflexology is just another modern fad, or yet another alternative therapy, given that there has been such a surge of interest in it during the last ten years or so. In fact, its origins are thought to be far more ancient than that. Native American Indians, for example, have practised a form of reflexology for hundreds of years. They have been aware of the exchange of energy from the earth through the feet, and how important it is that there are no blockages in the feet to impede the movement of energy.

There is other evidence to suggest that reflexology is an ancient practice. An Egyptian tomb mural depicts reflexologists at work. The mural, in the tomb of Ankhmahor, a famous physician of the day and dating back to about 2300 BC, illustrates what appears to be reflexology treatments being performed on both hands and feet.

Medicine was highly developed in Egypt in pharaonic times. The human body was studied in great detail and there is evidence that sophisticated surgical procedures were carried out. In Ankhmahor's tomb other murals give us an insight into the state of medicine at the time. Six murals depict circumcision, childbirth, dentistry, pharmacology, embalming and reflexology. The inclusion of reflexology amongst such prime practices shows how highly the therapy was valued.

And interestingly, inscribed in hieratic characters (a form of hieroglyphics favoured by priests in ancient Egypt) above the pictography are the patient's words: 'Do not let it be painful.' The practitioner replies, 'I shall act so you praise me,' sentiments which can be considered just as appropriate in today's practice of reflexology as they were then.

So how might reflexology have spread? During the Ptolemy dynasty, 323-80 BC, the great Alexandria library was established. This was mainly devoted to Greek texts, but also preserved large stores of Egyptian papyrus scrolls. It is very likely that scholars from Alexandria carried the knowledge of reflexology from Egypt, via Arabia, to Greece. Later, after the Roman conquest, it migrated further through Europe. Not much is known about reflexology during the following centuries, until Benvenuto Cellini, the great sixteenth-century Florentine sculptor, used strong pressure on his fingers and toes to relieve pain anywhere in his body, a method which echoes reflexology's practices.

Confidence in reflexology and other 'hands-on' therapies was for a time weakened in the Western world when at the end of the sixteenth century two Dutch spectacle makers, Hans and Zacharias Janssen, developed the microscope. A new visual world was thus opened up for the medical profession and medicine became more scientific. Doctors had confidence in what they could see rather than what they could not fully understand; a practice which is very much in evidence today despite the growth of complementary medicine in the West. With the development of safer and more effective anaesthesia in the nineteenth century, surgical procedures also became more intrusive – any organ not functioning properly was likely to be removed.

Dr William Fitzgerald (1872–1942), an American ear, nose and throat specialist, is the forefather of reflexology as we know it today. In 1902 he was studying in Vienna when the German physician Dr Alfonse Cornelius published his book, *Pressure Points – Their Origin and Significance*. This book was based on Cornelius's own experience during massage sessions while recovering from an infection. During the massage he could recognize reflex responses to pressure and, in conjunction with the masseur, identified and charted the pressure points. There was support for this theory from other physicians in Germany and some introduced the technique of reflex massage into their practice.

Dr Fitzgerald may or may not have been aware of this discovery while he was in Vienna, but since medical circles are small, he probably was. He returned to the United States and practised as the senior ear, nose and throat surgeon at St Francis' Hospital, in Hartford, Connecticut.

It is on record that in 1909 he conceived the notion of 'zone therapy'. By putting pressure on various parts of the hands, fingers and feet he found that a numbing effect would occur in another area. Dr Fitzgerald advocated the use of instruments to bring about this numbing effect; for example he would attach clothes pegs on the tips of fingers, apply rubber bands around the fingers or ask patients to grip combs in their hands. This allowed him to do minor ear, nose and throat surgery with little or no anaesthesia.

Based on the results of his research, together with prior knowledge he had gained in Europe, Dr Fitzgerald divided the body into ten theoretical zones, five on either side of the midline, terminating in the fingers and toes (see diagram on p.31). His theory stated that there was an energetic link throughout each zone. For instance, if the big toe on the right foot is being massaged, the effect of the massage would be felt throughout that whole long-itudinal zone, reaching up to the head and down to the right thumb.

Although Dr Fitzgerald's fellow doctors agreed that 'zone therapy' was profoundly effective, they found the technique too time-consuming and unorthodox to adopt it extensively. So Dr Fitzgerald turned to natural therapists as recipients of his knowledge. There was one colleague, Dr Jo Selby Riley, who was an eager convert to this new practice. He charted his findings of reflex areas in the feet, hands, ears and head in minute detail and wrote a number of published books and treatises on the subject.

However, the true matriarch of zone therapy was Eunice Ingham (1897–1974) who worked as a massage therapist for Dr Riley in St Petersburg, Florida. She adopted the name 'reflexology' for the therapy and concentrated her working field to the feet. Instead of using the techniques for relief of pain she adapted the pressure so that it stimulated and healed. Like Dr Fitzgerald, she shared her knowledge with chiropodists, naturopaths, masseurs and physiotherapists, as well as teaching patients the technique for treating themselves, their family and friends.

Eunice Ingham wrote four books on reflexology. The best known, *Stories the Feet Can Tell*, is still a popular and fascinating read. She was a great teacher, travelling all over the United States, assisted by her nephew Dwight C. Byers, and later his sister, Eusbia Messenger, RN. The former is still one of the leading teachers in America and worldwide.

This all sounds a great success story, but as a recognized therapy reflexology did not have an easy birth. The medical establishment at the time appeared to have felt threatened by it and it was dismissed as 'quackery'. In a number of American states the Medical Board of Examiners prosecuted therapists for practising medicine without a licence. As recently as 1968 Eunice Ingham was charged with this offence, though the charges were withdrawn before reaching court. It was some years before the therapy was recognized as having any value by orthodox medicine, and even now it is still not universally accepted by medical practitioners.

Doreen Bailey was the pioneer of the therapy in Britain. After training with Eunice Ingham in the United States, she returned to the UK in 1966 to open her own school, the Bailey School of Reflexology. Her pupils are now practising and teaching her method in Britain and abroad. In 1978 Bailey wrote a book called *Reflexology Today* which gives a clear and concise explanation of reflexology and her experiences with it. It is a valuable text.

Universal acceptance has been almost as difficult to achieve in Britain as in the United States. The British are notoriously cautious about new ideas and reflexology was no exception. Now, more than two decades after Mrs Bailey started her work in Britain, there are many schools providing courses. As demand for complementary therapies increases the standard of teaching and course content is being looked at more closely to ensure that well-trained therapists are available to the public.

There are also various professional bodies which give advice regarding the training requirements, curriculum content and standards of teaching in an endeavour to ensure quality tuition. Accredited courses normally last at least nine months on a part-time basis, incorporating theory, practice and home study, which is completed by a practical and written examination. There are many introductory courses which give a student a taster of the therapy. These courses are useful for those who are considering further training but want to be sure it is right for them. Others find them valuable to acquire enough knowledge to give treatments to family and friends.

Sometimes people who have trained as reflexologists set up private practices working from home. Others offer their services voluntarily to hospices. Many therapists work in natural health clinics, sports centres and beauty salons and some GPs are referring patients with chronic conditions to reflexologists.

The use of reflexology in hospitals varies. Several have introduced the therapy in obstetrics and some in intensive care units – there is no uniform policy about reflexology as yet, but the new 'enlightenment' about its use is encouraging. Some nurses take a course on their own initiative and a few are sponsored by their health authority and incorporate reflexology into their nursing practice.

The English National Board for Nursing, Midwifery and Health Visiting, which sets the nursing curriculum, is now offering a post-graduate course in the philosophies of complementary therapies and will include an introduction to reflexology. It is a ten-week postgraduate course at Durham and Teeside College of Health for nurses, but also open to general practitioners and people who are in the caring services. The course is designed to heighten their awareness of the philosophy of complementary therapies so that they can have an understanding of what these therapies are, before referring.

While reflexology tends to be overshadowed in this country by the 'big four' complementary therapies – acupuncture, osteopathy, chiropractic and homeopathy – in Denmark reflexology is the most common complementary treatment used. A Gallup poll carried out in 1993 showed that 39 per cent of the people questioned had some experience of reflexology. The Danish Reflexologist Association has done some exciting research projects, including a study on reflexology in the workplace.

One particularly interesting project started three years ago when the Post and Telegraph Authorities offered their staff a new type of personal health care: they employed in-house reflexologists to treat staff out of work hours. Conditions treated included back pain, muscular tension, skeletal problems, headache/migraine, stomach/intestinal and hormonal imbalances. Many of these conditions treated are stress-related. Statistical proof showed that during the time of the reflexology treatments there was a great reduction in the number of working days lost through sick leave. The saving on sick pay was much greater than the reflexologist's salary, but more important was the increased feeling of well-being and motivation among the employees and their appreciation that something was being done to improve the quality of their working life.

The potential cost-effectiveness of reflexology when used to deal with absenteeism in the workplace has also been demonstrated by a recent study of 28 staff seen within the Worcester hospitals using reflexology treatments. The study was undertaken by Anne Jordan, a complementary therapist specializing in reflexology, aromatherapy and visualization. After six treatment sessions the twenty-two women and six men assessed experienced a variety of responses. Seventeen found that they experienced a significant improvement in quality of life and pain reduction. Nineteen noticed increased mobility. Sixteen noticed increased energy levels and twenty had a more positive psyche. Every single therapee reported a degree of change in some aspect of their life.

Anne Jordan concludes that reflexology is a cost-effective treatment for those companies and institutions thinking of benefits for their staff and coping with absenteeism, one of the main problems in industry and the Health Service. The effect on staff morale, of the availability of a therapist is a very positive one, even when staff pay for treatments. In an ideal situation the treatments should be funded by the institution. The positive effects of this would result in a happier working environment and far fewer staff on the sick list.

She also points out that according to the Confederation of British Industry, UK employers lose £13 billion annually due to sickness absence. At the CBI conference on absenteeism at work it was stated that, with an absence reduction programme a one per cent reduction should be achievable in the first year. This would represent a saving of £60,000 for a 500-strong company in direct costs alone (Occupational Health Review May/June 1993). British management places too much emphasis on controlling absence as a disciplinary issue and not enough on the health aspects of sickness absence.

Another similarly slanted project was carried out by a Danish health department with home helps. In the six-month period during which a reflexologist was employed there were less than 2,499 sick leave hours taken compared to the same period in a previous year. The big advantage was that staff could get treatment immediately after acute illness. This was considered the reason why no long-term sick leave was required during the reflexology period. This particular health department has now employed a reflexologist full-time for the common good of their entire staff.

China, too, is a country where reflexology is used extensively in preventative health rather than in curing dis-ease. The Ancient Chinese philosophy has always been to pay their doctors to keep the people well and not when dis-ease takes hold. Reflexology as a is valued as an economic, safe and effective method for assuring the general well-being of the nation. In China reflexology is taught on television and by video programmes for family education as well as in teaching schools for professionals.

Recently Suzanne attended the China Preventive Medicine Association conference in Beijing where the subject was foot reflexology. The use of the therapy is widespread in China and in the area where it is practised most extensively the medical expenses have fallen by one third. The users' health improved as did their longevity. From her own experience she can understand this as the therapees in the London centre, in which she practises, who had reflexology treatments over a period of time found that they did not require the same number of painkillers or anti-spasmodic drugs that they used to take, and did not get as many infections requiring antibiotics as they had prior to treatment. All this would reflect on the health costs and would balance to an extent the expenditure on therapists.

Other countries, not already mentioned, where the therapy is rapidly gaining recognition include United States of America, Germany, Holland, the Scandinavian countries, Greece, Israel, Malaysia, Taiwan, Australia, New Zealand and South Africa. There is, though, still much to be done. So to promote reflexology around the world the International Council for Reflexology was founded in September 1990 to hold a conference bi-annually in a different country each time. This serves to spread the knowledge regarding research and other aspects related to the therapy, and most important creates a link between therapists around the world and in turn strengthens the understanding between nations. And in September 1994 the first European Conference of Reflexology was held in Newcastle University with delegates from 12 countries.

All these recent developments show how reflexology is being acknowledged as having a mainstream place in complementary therapy and how there is a wonderful exchange of ideas among therapists throughout the world. Reflexology is no longer 'wacky'. Its advantages are beginning to be accepted by many.

Chapter Two
How Does it Work ?

In 1948, the World Health Organisation defined health as '. . . a state of complete physical, mental and social well-being and not merely the absence of disease or infirmity.' We prefer the sentiments of the Lady of the Lamp, British nurse Florence Nightingale, who is remembered for her work during the Crimean War (1853–6).

She believed that one had to participate in the maintenance of health. In her words: 'Health is not only to be well, but to use well every power we have.' Our understanding of this definition is that you need to pay attention to what your body is telling you and if possible respond to it. When you are feeling really tired perhaps allow yourself to have some early nights if you can. When you need a break take time out if at all feasible. These are simple strategies to avoid a state of dis-ease developing, to clear your distracted mind and to help your body adapt to what is going on around it.

To us this definition of health is a much more useful one because in *The Reflexology Partnership* we try to illustrate how reflexology can be used as a means of realizing your true potential and how it can allow you to tune in to your body's messages. The means justifies the end rather than the end justifying the means.

Florence Nightingale was enlightened enough to realize that being physically impaired is no handicap to wholeness. And to us, wholeness is what reflexology is all about. It treats the whole person, not just sorting out a particular symptom.

Reflexology is a holistic therapy since the effect of the treatment is experienced on the physical, mental, emotional and spiritual levels. It is a method of assisting the body in its self-healing process through the medium of touch. It is an engagement between two people which allows an energetic exchange to take place.

We believe reflexology is a safe, simple, drug-free way of maintaining health and general well-being. Communication can be made with the whole person by touching the feet alone. There does not have to be any other form of communication. It need not involve a series of questions and answers. The feet do the talking.

A therapist can feel the constantly changing levels of the body's energy in the feet. The tone of the skin and the tissues can show whether a person is tired or not. Feet also show feelings of well-being. People's state of being can change like the weather. Our emotions can flow through the four seasons in one day!

The feet are a barometer of your state of being at any particular moment. And through touch alone a therapist can respond sensitively to what the feet are saying.

The joy of the therapy, too, is that where relevant it combines well with both orthodox medicine and other natural therapies. It is truly 'complementary' because it can so readily be combined in this way. If you take a person who is being treated with drugs for arthritis, reflexology can be combined with the orthodox treatment to help resolve any underlying cause.

So what exactly does reflexology involve? It is a type of foot massage based on the belief that our bodies are reflected in microcosm in our feet. This miniature representation is also found in other areas including our hands, ears, tongues, backs and even internally, for example, in our large intestines.

But how the sense of touch through reflexology is able to work is a question that is difficult to answer. Today there are several theories as to how reflexology works and we cannot be definite about which theory is correct.

The zone theory was the fundamental concept of how reflexology worked. Zones are a three-dimensional linear subdivision of the body in theoretical sections. Imagine the body being cut lengthways between each toe and then being glued together again. It is as if each toe is a beacon-like terminal at the end of the zone.

So it follows that there are ten zones, five on the right side of the body and five on the left. The right side of the body is reflected in the right foot and vice versa. This division is also applicable to the hands with the division coming between each finger, and the zones running up to the head.

There is no physical manifestation of these zones, yet Dr Fitzgerald (who conceived the notion of zone therapy in 1909 and who was the forefather of reflexology as we know it today) observed that there was an energetic connection between all the organs, muscles, nerves, blood supply and tissue within each zone. That is how working in a zone triggers an energetic effect throughout that zone. For instance, by working in zone one on the right foot, energy is activated throughout that zone in the body, for example, a part of the reproductive organs, bladder, right side of the spine, the throat and so on.

The big toe is interesting because all five zones of the head are represented in miniature, almost a three dimensional passport photo superimposed on your big toes.

Dr Selby Riley identified eight horizontal zones, but today

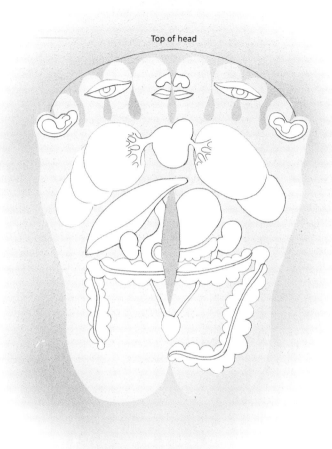

Top of head

reflexologists identify four anatomical divisions in the body: the shoulder girdle, the diaphragm, the waistline and the pelvic girdle. See diagram opposite.

Thinking about the structure and shape of the foot, it is comprehensible to identify how these contour/defining lines were drawn. This 'grid' is a useful framework as an aid in identifying the location of all the body parts as found in the feet.

We feel that this book is not the place to discuss the reflex areas of the foot in detail. We merely seek to explain in a broad sense what reflexology's basic principles are, so that you, the reader, can make an informed choice of whether reflexology is the therapy for you.

As you can see from the diagram of the feet with the body superimposed on their outline, in its simplest sense, the head, which houses the brain, is reflected in the toes, and so these are concerned with our thinking processes. Moving down the body, the chest is involved with expression of feeling, while the upper abdomen is concerned with how we function with ourselves and other people in work situations and life generally.

The pelvic area is related to our creativity and close relationships with the give and take of family life. The heel area is mobility, drive, direction and security.

With the development of scientific technology that basis of zone therapy has been explored, elaborated upon and taken further.

We believe one of the most exciting new theories has recently been put forward by a biologist specialising in how the brain works. At a meeting of the Reflexologists' Association in 1991 Roger Coghill explained how he believed that the body's healing process is activated in the brain. Health, he observed, was an old Anglo Saxon term meaning wholeness or completeness – so that when healing takes place the person is becoming whole or complete again. In this case, it is not the therapist who 'does' the healing but the therapee. It is the therapist who assists in creating the conditions necessary to activate the healing process in the brain.

During normal wear and tear the body loses about 500 million cells a day. The body restores these cells by a process of cell division

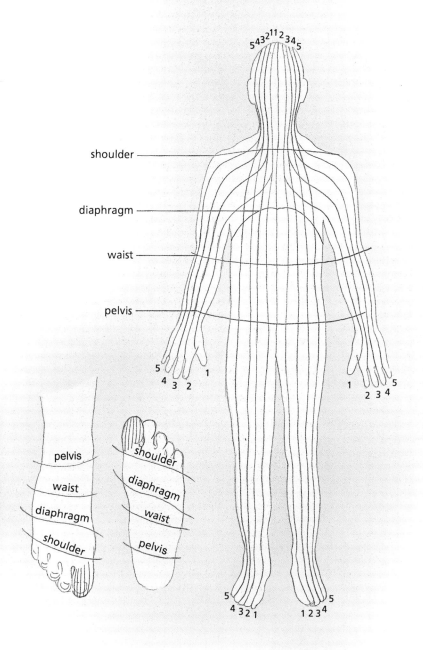

known as mitosis. The miracle of mitosis is that each new cell is a clone containing a copy of the DNA in the nucleus of the parent cell. Coghill believes that the brain triggers this action of mitosis during sound sleep. Scientists used to think that nerve impulses stimulated this process but it has been acknowledged that this cannot be so since the speed of nerve conduction is not fast enough.

The stimulus may therefore be electro-magnetic – as fast as radio waves – which is the speed of light! Coghill was one of the first to point out that the brain is built like a radio transmission set: it is divided into two halves or hemispheres, joined at the base by a band of some 30,000 cell fibres. The cells in one half are sometimes positive, sometimes negative. This polarity alternates all the time as electrons (ions) pulse rapidly from one side to the other. To assist this activity the hemispheres oscillate like jellies. Through this process radio frequency energy is broadcast to the cells of the body.

Extra low frequency brainwaves (human E.L.F.) were discovered in 1929 by Dr Hans Berger. These waves are interesting as they can penetrate the entire body. This radio broadcast system has always existed in nature, but until recently biologists tended to think only in terms of chemical effects. Technology now is able to allow these waves to be recorded and measured.

Since the feet are the most distant part of the body from the brain, Coghill's researches have proposed that the electromagnetic signals transmitted to them are the strongest. He proposes this because the motor/sensory areas in the brain relevant to the feet are closest together, hence carry the strongest charges, and this leads in turn to the strongest signals.

It follows then, that during a reflexology treatment on the feet, signals are returned to this same highly charged area in the brain. Here they are processed and stimuli are then discharged throughout the nerve cells in the outer covering of the brain (cortex), called association fibres, and then transferred by the central nervous system to the body.

It is an exciting theory and if Coghill is right, then a whole new insight into the way our bodies work has been identified. In our experience people often remark that following a reflexology treatment they sleep more soundly than they have for a long time, even years. This is interesting as it seems to affirm Roger Coghill's explanation as to how reflexology assists in the regeneration process. When people sleep soundly they are letting the repair work of mitosis take place as it should.

Another theory of reflexology is based on the assumption that health improves when the body can regularly experience a state of relaxation. Putting it simply, when this specific massage is applied to the feet, ideally a state of relaxation is created which consequently facilitates the body's innate self-regulating healing process.

The effect of reflexology is to re-establish the body's natural rhythm. This releases stress and tension, allowing blood to circulate more efficiently to all the cells of the body and to assist in the excretion of waste material. The process can assist in pain relief and bring about a sense of well-being, or homeostasis.

This term was coined by W.B. Cannon, a physiologist in the 1930s, to describe 'the various physiologic arrangements which serve to restore the normal state, once it has been disturbed.'

The cells of the body are surrounded by extracellular fluid and for the cells to function efficiently, the composition of this 'internal

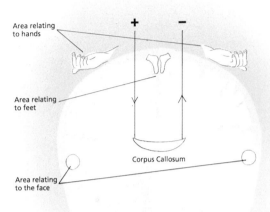

Area relating to hands

Area relating to feet

Area relating to the face

Corpus Callosum

sea' needs to remain constant. This state of constancy is called homeostasis. This is a term frequently used in relation to the effect of reflexology yet many people are not truly clear as to its meaning.

Reflexology can be used to restore homeostasis. When the normal rhythm of breathing is disturbed it is a sign that homeostasis is being damaged. When a person is stressed, for example, that is, feeling mentally, emotionally or physically strained or tense, the normal breathing pattern is lost. Frequently in this state people either breathe superficially or hyperventilate. The effect of this is to alter the chemical balance of the internal sea so the body's cells cannot function optimally. This inefficient breathing method grossly disturbs the exchange of oxygen and carbon dioxide. This upsets the acid/alkaline balance in their bodies.

Carbon dioxide helps to keep people calm. It controls the diameter of the blood vessels supplying the brain. During hyperventilation the flow of blood to the brain is impeded. This can cause a feeling of light-headedness, anxiety, tiredness, weakness, chest pain, loss of concentration, disturbed sleep, digestive disorders and depression. On the other hand, too much carbon dioxide in the blood makes it too acid. This can cause headache, confusion and eventually coma.

In this state uric acid may collect and become deposited in the toes creating a sensation which feels like crystals under the skin. These clear during the balancing process of the reflexology treat- ment. We have observed that people who have endured ongoing stress, often for a long time, will have these crystals primarily in the toes. Before these crystals begin to form we have also felt areas of what can only be described as a slight impeding of an energetic flow which shoot away from under the finger when pressure is applied. The therapee can feel something akin to a tiny energetic jolt followed by a feeling of release, a restoring of balance. It is this balance which is the key to maintaining homeostasis and a balance that reflexology can restore.

There are therapists who believe that some of the beneficial effects of reflexology are caused by massaging the meridians in the feet. In acupuncture meridians are basically thought of as linking pathways which carry our vital energies through the body. There are twelve main meridians either side of the body, each related to specific organs, such as the heart, liver and stomach. There are six main meridians running through the feet. They are the liver, spleen, pancreas, stomach, gall bladder and kidney meridians.

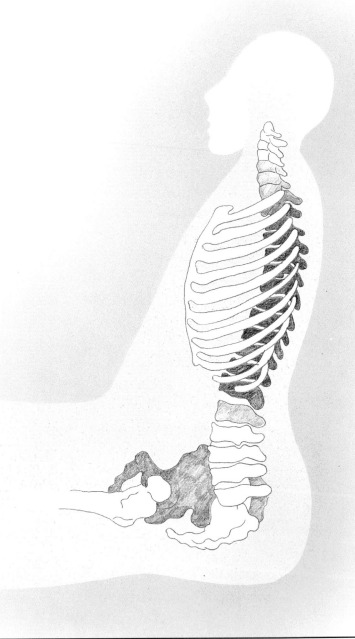

During reflexology being aware of the acupuncture meridians and the organs they relate to can enrich treatment.

The concept of holography is another theory. A holograph is a three-dimensional picture and one essential element of holography is that the part reflects the whole. According to Helle Johannessen, a scientist writing for the Danish Reflexologists Association, the principle of the part reflecting the whole may explain the existence of reflex zones in the feet and the fact that there is an effect in the body when the feet are treated. Using a map of the feet with a projection of the entire body, reflexology is based on the principle of the part reflecting the whole.

Johannessen goes on to explain that the connection is structural and consists of a correlation between the overall pattern of the feet and the overall pattern of the body. The feet and the body are both interpreted as an expression of a common organizing pattern for this particular individual. When manipulating the pattern in the feet, the common organizing pattern is altered, thereby influencing the pattern in the entire body.

This is illustrated when you give a treatment to someone with a chest infection. You can feel a sensation of congestion in the ball of the foot which is the related part. Or when someone has damaged his or her knee that injury can also be felt immediately as pain in the related area of the foot.

Of course, for some people accepting a therapy without a definite and scientific explanation of how it works is very difficult. They may accept that the body has tremendous powers to heal itself if they cut a finger and then see it heal, or if they bruise an arm badly and see the bruise disappear. But they find it difficult to accept that the healing powers of the body can go further than that. And then there are the sceptics who believe reflexology works by the placebo effect. The word placebo is a medieval Latin phrase which was used in vespers for the 'Placebo in Domino in Regione Vivorum', which translated means 'I shall please the Lord in the land of the living', from *placere* to please.

A placebo is a substance used as a medicine without an active drug, administered to a patient who believes it to be an active drug. The 'drugless' medicine is given to humour the patient or to effect a cure by changing the patient's psychological attitude by this deception. When it works it is called the placebo effect. It has even been proved in research that the more faith the doctor has in the drugs he prescribes the more effective those drugs are likely to be.

When a child hurts himself a maternal 'Mummy will kiss it better' frequently works wonders. It is your child. You are concerned and you are putting all your energy into making the hurt better. It is an energetic exchange.

So the sceptics say when a person really believes in the powers of reflexology that alone works wonders. But if a patient believes a treatment is proving beneficial, and enjoys an hour of undivided attention, does it really matter how it works, the strength is that it does.

So why the feet? While recognizing the variety of responsive sites in the body, in this book, we are focusing particularly on the feet, not only for simplicity, but also because the feet are also considered the most receptive sites for massage.

There is some conflict about using the word massage when talking about reflexology. It is thought that the hand actions used during a reflexology session are dissimilar to those used in a full body massage.

Yet looking through the English dictionaries we cannot find a word which more adequately describes the action of reflexology than the Collins Concise English Dictionary definition of massage as 'the act of kneading, rubbing etc. parts of the body to promote circulation, suppleness and relaxation'. 'Etc.', perhaps, describes the massage movements used in reflexology which are specially adapted to suit the structure of the hands and feet. These extremities are well designed tools for action, expression, movement and weight-bearing. They are also brilliantly receptive tools for communication by touch through the means of massage.

In reflexology treatments are carried out on the feet and hands primarily. Treating the hands is beneficial, they are easily accessible for self-treatment and useful when foot treatment is contra-indicated, such as the feet being too ticklish, too painful or when the skin is so fragile it could rupture on contact. Some therapists treat both feet and hands in one session and find this combination effective.

The hands, though, form a more intimate communication and care is needed when they are being considered for treatment. There are some explanations as to why this may be so. The tips of the fingers contain specialized nerve endings which are involved in the mystery of human touch. So there is a great increase and magnification of what happens during touch. For some people having their hands done is too intimate an experience.

Lovers hold hands and at times that can be an exquisite feeling. It is also just pleasant, comfortable and nurturing. The hands can be used to reach out to others. The hands and arms are used to hug people and this action is usually reserved for people close to us.

From our experience treatment on the feet has been found to be more effective. The feet are larger and there is space for detail and movement. Feet replicate the body's shape, making it is easier to identify where energy flow is disturbed. The effect of the earth's gravitational pull results in areas of congestion showing up more clearly in the feet and at times there is almost a feeling of sediment having settled in the feet.

We find that therapees become more receptive to treatment when their feet are being treated because they are reclining, their body weight is supported and they relax more freely which allows energetic replenishment to take place. They are also not in such intimate contact with the therapist which they could find disturbing.

Foot reflexology can be useful for so many people as feet are easily accessible. If you are a wheelchair user you can have reflexology while still sitting in it, if you wish. Even if you have no sensation in your feet, reflexology can still be beneficial because the effects of a reflexology foot massage can be felt throughout the body, including the mental and spiritual levels. Our hands, too, fit around the feet so easily and comfortably – as if they were designed for that purpose.

Chapter 3
Touch and the Reflexology Partnership

'The communications we transmit through touch constitute the most powerful means of establishing human relationships, the foundation of experience.'

Ashley Montagu
Touching. The Human Significance of the Skin. 1986 Preface XV.

Touch can be life-giving or life-destroying. It is an open dialogue where intentions are more difficult to camouflage than they would be when you communicate through words.

Through reflexology life-giving touch brings nurturing feelings of comfort, security, trust, acceptance and relaxation. Touch that generates feelings of withdrawal, physical tensing of the body, pain, rejection and uneasiness will not nurture. Touch communicates our intentions more clearly than words. As we live through our bodies, we listen more attentively to the messages given by touch than we often do to messages given by words. Words can be easier to ignore than sensations of pleasure or pain, for example.

Touching is something instinctive which we do all the time yet we seldom stop to consider how complex this activity is. Of the five senses, touch is the first to develop in both the human and animal embryo. A six-week-old foetus has been shown to respond to touch before its eyes and ears have developed. The developing ovum is composed of three primitive layers which form the different parts of the growing baby. The outer layer, the ectoderm, forms the central nervous system and extends to develop the body skin, hair, nails and teeth.

The foundation for understanding the effect of all 'hands-on' therapies is to realize that the skin is the largest sensory organ of the body. Its role is vital and incredibly complex. Skin has many functions. It protects the body as a waterproof envelope. Another function is reducing our temperature by sweating in a hot environment. Specialized nerve endings in the skin send signals that the brain identifies as touch, pain, pressure, heat and cold. It can be said to provide the external nervous system while the central nervous system is the buried part. No wonder that when we are under emotional strain or pressure physical symptoms may appear, for example, our hair loses its gloss, our skin goes blotchy or develops a rash and when we are under very serious pressure our hair can even fall out.

How and why does this happen? The outer layer of the skin, the epidermis, is the seat of touch. The cells contain millions of sensory receptors which transport the information by the nerves via the spinal cord to the brain. Here decisions are made to activate physical or emotional responses. Touch can also be a major form of communication between people – a silent language.

Many years ago, Suzanne's husband, a surgeon, had a deep-seated malignant growth removed by a colleague and close friend. After the operation the surgeon had to break the news to her that her husband would not live much longer. Clearly this was a distressing situation for them both. Although in a state of shock she can remember thinking that if only he had felt able to put a hand on her shoulder she might have felt less isolated. Perhaps his own pain was so great that he could not respond.

But touch can offer comfort without any words being spoken. For example, its value has been recognized and used creatively in the Pat a Dog schemes run by some hospitals for elderly people and those with chronic or terminal illness. Suzanne's previous neighbours had an affable gun dog, Bodger, who once a week used to drag his mistress enthusiastically up the street to the local hospital where he did a ward round presenting himself to be patted by those patients who enjoyed the contact. It was a mutual admiration society, Bodger basking in the attention and the patients being nourished by the soothing action of gently stroking his silky coat and the dog's loving appreciation of the contact. Yet there are many of us who underestimate the value of touch even though so many expressions in common usage acknowledge the importance of touch in everyday life.

How often do we say 'I'll get in touch' even if we are going to use the phone as a form of contact! Someone may have done you an unexpected kindness and you feel 'touched' by their action. Things may be getting out of control in our lives and we feel a need 'to take a grip' on ourselves. We 'hold fast' to our beliefs and habits of a lifetime. Possibly you have felt the need to give yourself 'a pat on the back' when you have achieved something difficult. We all have our 'touchy' or 'prickly' acquaintances. How many times in our lives do we say that we feel as if someone has trampled all over us? This is often said when someone has been through a very difficult or trying time that needed all their energy to survive a threat.

Touch has wide-ranging permutations in our language and it also has wide-ranging effects when used in reflexology. It can be beneficial and promote feelings of warmth and well-being or it can be intrusive and invasive. We truly believe that the therapist must appreciate the value of touch and consequently must not abuse it. In reflexology the quality of the therapist's touch is paramount and it is important that it is acceptable to you and answers your need.

Therapists must be aware and must respond to what the therapee is experiencing. We are concerned about reports that therapees have experienced severe pain in a reflexology session.

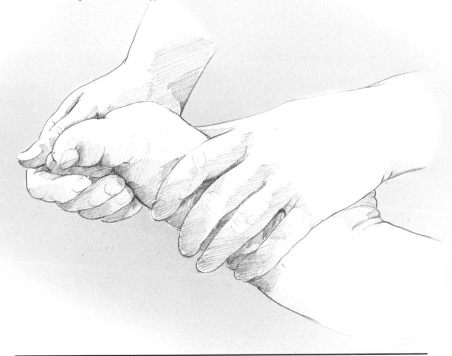

Pain is a warning signal and must not be ignored. Treatment is a two-way flow in unison. Therapists should stop and think about the effects of a reflexology treatment. Therapees all have individual needs and the amount and type of touch should be tailored to suit those individual needs.

Suzanne spoke to a man with cerebral palsy the other day who related his experience with reflexology in the past. His ability to communicate is limited by his disablement yet he managed to convey to the therapist that the pain he felt during the session was so severe it made him cry. But the therapist still continued with the treatment and he felt no benefit at all afterwards. Quite rightly he will not return to that therapist for further treatment. However, some people with cerebral palsy use more energy in daily life than the average person due to spasm, possible communication and mobility problems and they really do benefit from sensitive, relaxing treatments which help to relieve spasm and enhance the body's regenerative process.

This observation is born out in a statement made on a computer by a 45-year-old woman with cerebral palsy. 'When I have reflexology I am nice and relaxed. And this all lasts for a few days. After a session I can walk better and I can straighten my knees when I am walking.'

A lot of what we do, as therapists as in the rest of life, can be learned and improves with practice. The reflexology session is dependent on the needs of the recipient. A session should not be based on a therapist's needs to see results, or to heal. A therapist has to forget his or her self and act selflessly by putting the therapee's needs before their own. When a therapist is with a person in this spirit, the spirit of an attendant, rather than as a director, the temptation to 'cure' or to show how to get rid of symptoms is diminished.

When the therapist takes on the role of director the temptation to take over increases. This temptation can be felt by the therapist and the therapee. The easy way to solve our problems is to ask someone to do it for us. This has been the approach in medicine with the doctor who can fix a problem. We go to the doctor in order to tell him or her our symptoms. By doing this we give the doctor the responsibility to fix us. We are all so used to this approach. When people have their feet done they often want to be told what to do, because this is the kind of relationship they have come to expect. Many practitioners are only too happy to assume a senior position and tell the person what to do. But this is not a partnership. It is essential that a therapist is aware of the inherent danger of sessions conducted in an atmosphere of domination and submission. Neither domination nor submission can occur when people are truly interacting together, equally contributing to the benefit of each other.

The very nature of a reflexology session, with one person sitting or reclining with bare feet, while the other is sitting upright with feet covered, places people who may have a tendency to want to control or want to submit in a vulnerable position. In a healing partnership both people co-operate together.

If a reflexologist has a need to see a change in a person's feet, symptoms or life pattern, then there is a barrier that prevents a true partnership forming. If change is desired that means the therapist is acting in a judgemental way. A reflexologist who equates improvement with success is constantly struggling to keep on winning and feeling good. If the therapist is looking for 'results' there is happiness when there is improvement, and distress when there is deterioration. This is unhealthy.

While you are in this mode of thinking you are imposing your view of how someone needs to be in order to please yourself. 'Ah,' you say, 'but it is for his own good.' If you are honest there is usually something in it for your own good. It could be said that wanting to help, or to heal, is worthy, as opposed to wanting to make money or be famous, but they are equal desires as they are based on satisfying a need. Even seekers of spiritual development, which is often portrayed as the noblest pursuit of all, can be motivated by need. This need can make them vulnerable and can end up in them being controlled by an unscrupulous guru.

Be aware of a therapist who has the need to take charge of you in order to 'make you better' because the underlying presupposition there is that you are not OK, and that the way you are does not work. But does not work for whom? You or the therapist? Ideally you should feel comfortable with your therapist as someone you can trust, is empathetic and non-judgemental. You should also feel comfortable with his or her touch.

Suzanne remembers some years ago, the relatives of a man who was disabled asking her to treat him as they thought it would be good for him. This was in her early days as a therapist, in her full flush of altruism, and in her concern for him in his disabled condition she visited him at home twice a week for some months. He enjoyed the company and found the treatment pleasurable as he did his dependence. As the months passed changes took place. His mobility and bladder control improved and pain subsided. The family was excited in the expectation of his doing his own shopping again. However, as far as he was concerned, this was the down side of the therapy and he found a variety of reasons why it was inappropriate for the treatment to continue.

Afterwards Suzanne heard that he had entered a residential home where he felt secure, supported and happy. It was a valuable lesson for Suzanne and she is grateful that she experienced it early in her career as a therapist. It made her respect the fact that for some people their dis-ease is their coping method and they do not want to change. Since then she does not treat anyone unless it has been their own decision to have reflexology treatments, that they understand the therapy and that they are prepared to accept any changes that may occur.

From a therapist's point of view it is reassuring knowing that the person they are treating has been motivated to experience reflexology and is aware that the process of change is within them not the therapist. Your motivation is the key to your process and you and the therapist are then working as a team.

By all means discuss your needs and goals with the therapist, who is the catalyst in the process of change. This sharing is an important part of the partnership. A sensitive therapist can identify your needs, to some extent, in your feet, yet you play an active part in this team approach and must feel free to comment as the treatment proceeds. If there is a degree, or form, of touch you do, or do not like just say so. You are not expected to play a passive role in this partnership.

A healing bond can develop when the therapist and therapee are in the roles of attendant and attended. The therapist in this role is not trying to 'do' anything for the person, but is responding to what the person needs for his or her comfort. This way a barter system does not operate and the therapist is attentive and aware.

A therapist who enjoys being with people and interacting freely has a headstart. The feeling of space and openness that is created when two people join in the reflexology partnership could be called freedom. This does not always happen but is the optimum condition for healing, in the sense of restoring the body's balance and facilitating change. In this state a person can see more clearly, understand their problems and take action.

In the reflexology partnership the quality of touch is adapted to the messages coming from the feet and the therapist endeavours to do this as best he or she can.

In their honesty the feet give off messages about the therapee's needs at the time. Subtle signs show early in the feet. If the therapist is not fully aware and present these nuances can be missed, and the flow of communication changed from one of ease and comfort to a state of distress. For example, a slight inversion of a foot is a sign that the person having reflexology is experiencing a difficult situation and it shows itself physically in the foot. The role of the therapist is to respond with understanding through touch. In response to touch the body's action is automatic and it is real. This is the natural coping mechanism and needs to be taken into consideration. You cannot think your way out of it. Your mind cannot control how your body reacts to touch. This language is learned through experience and ideally, a therapist is a sensitive human being. This quality will provide a firm base on which technical know-how will be built. This open communication does not flourish when therapist and therapee are not involved in a partnership. That is why the attitudes between patient and therapist are paramount to the progress of treatment sessions. There must be a respect in that relationship. When you do reflexology you are not only involved in massage you are also directly touching a person's vital energy and it can have a great impact on that person's life. The state of the therapist's own energy is also an important factor in this exchange. As we mentioned earlier each one of us is made up of energy vibrating at various frequencies.

While we strongly believe that a good two-way relationship between a therapist and therapee is essential for the healing process to begin, we also have to point out that within this framework each relationship is individual. Each therapist has a different personality, a different touch and way of working, and certainly each therapee has a different personality and different needs. There are some people who say, well I went to a reflexologist and she did not do anything. I did not feel any better. I did not feel as though anything had happened at all. There are people who feel they need to be beaten with a stick almost. And if they have not felt this pain they do not feel they have gained by the treatment. Some therapists have an eloquent touch carrying on a conversation with you through your feet. Others have skilled mechanical touch which is concerned with fixing things. The touch of each person is as unique as their fingerprints. Blind people can recognize their friends by their touch. It is very useful that there are so many choices of touch in the field of reflexology so the client can choose that which suits them. Some people find stimulating touch pleasing. Other people respond to a gentle touch. Also the quality of touch appropriate for each person will vary from one treatment to another according to how the person is feeling at the time.

As we said earlier a perceptive therapist will recognize the needs of the client and adapt their method of treating accordingly. The therapee is in the strong position of having the choice. If you do not feel comfortable with the quality of the touch you are receiving you should discuss this with your therapist. If they are not able to adapt then you can make a change. Therapists should never take this switching personally as we are all aware of the positive and negative poles in human relationships which is all part of the richness of life. We have all had people who you see once and never see again. That is their prerogative and one wishes them well. The freedom of choice is the important element here, not our personal feelings.

Some years ago Suzanne was covering the practices of two of her colleagues who were away on holiday. It was fascinating to note that each therapist had attracted very different types of clients. Suzanne also realized at this time that the people who came to her for treatments were different again. It was interesting as this difference was not limited to the areas where the practices were situated. Some patients had travelled from long distances to reach the therapist. It must have all been to do with this magnetic attraction which is so strong in human interaction but one does not give it much consideration. Yet it is important that it be recognized and respected.

Do not give up the idea of treatments just because one experience has not been satisfying for you. All therapists are aware that the therapee's feeling of comfort with the touch is of prime importance in their getting the most benefit from a treatment, and that if a feeling of partnership is not going to develop then the right strategy for both of you is to make a change. When a feeling of partnership does exist the level of touch is comforting. The energetic exchange which has occurred brings about a change in both therapist and therapee and they are both uplifted. Through touch chemical changes will have taken place, fine-tuning the homeostatic process and restoring joie de vivre.

CHAPTER 4
HOW REFLEXOLOGY CAN HELP YOU

If you are thinking of experiencing reflexology you do need to be aware that there is a difference between this art, based on touch alone, and the medical science where a patient is expecting to be told what is wrong with him and what medicine or steps he needs to take to be cured. Each has its strengths and weaknesses and the important thing is to know when each is appropriate.

We believe that sensitive reflexology can be used in conjunction with medical treatment to enhance the healing process. There are times when reflexology alone can restore.

It allows a person to function in peak form and in this way it is good for helping to prevent dis-ease. For example, a person suffering from many colds may be becoming generally overloaded and their immune response is weakened.

Reflexology helps to increase the energy needed to throw off infections such as colds.

Many people with all manner of problems find reflexology useful. Nevertheless, we feel uncomfortable with the plethora of books listing an A–Z of conditions that reflexology can alleviate. From our point of view the art of reflexology is not about treating a particular condition but treating the person with an imbalance in the body's vital energy that is created by unrelieved stress, environmental factors, drinking too much alcohol, inappropriate diet, and a long list of other factors. This imbalance may bring about physical dis-ease which manifests itself in many forms.

Reflexology puts you in touch with the inner strength we all have that allows you to approach things positively. It develops a sense of self-worth, confidence in your own ability and faith in your own actions.

Reflexology does not dwell on a particular symptom. Through reflexology thoughts and emotions can be revealed and people understand why situations have occurred when they might never have understood before. So much discomfort with mental and emotional causes manifests itself in physical symptoms. During the time Eilish had her frozen shoulder she realized it was because she was not free to speak and do as she wanted. She could not be herself and this showed in her physical self.

Rather than reflexology being used to deal with one particular symptom, it can be used to balance once more the body's natural equilibrium and in this way restoration and repair can take place. The reflexology partnership is a form of communication between people with the language of touch. It can help relax the whole body and mind. It can remove congestion and blockages from energy pathways. It can improve blood circulation and aid the normalization of organ and gland function and consequently bring about balance and a feeling of well-being. Quite often reflexology can help people start a change in their life which helps them heal and live again in harmony. One woman who had ME told Suzanne that during the course of reflexology treatments she realized that although she had ME it was not only the illness that was making her life unhappy. It was also she felt that she was in the wrong job, and had the wrong partner that was causing her unhappiness. Suzanne heard from her later and discovered that she had met another man and was working in a different environment. Her life was now quite different and she acknowledged ME and paced her life accordingly.

Bringing about a change can be useful in dealing with unhealthy stress. When there is too much input for us to cope with we become stressed. Then we are inefficient, and even though we can bypass the distress signals it shows in our results.

A certain amount of stress can be healthy. A certain amount is good for you. It keeps you alive and it keeps you alert. Stress excites athletes before a race or a rugby match. After the event they relax and return to their usual mode of being. This is what is called the fright, fight or flight response.

What is stressful for one person may not be stressful for another. What is stressful at one time may not be stressful at another. But when that state of stress, or over-stimulation, becomes constant, when you are always on red alert which can lead to 'burn out', you ask too much of your body and it cannot function efficiently.

On the other hand, when there is no exhilarating stress, the state of 'fizzle out' develops when there is no spark which makes you feel alive. Life appears to be just a series of dull routines. In both these situations reflexology can help equalize these extremes and bring about a sense of equanimity.

Stress triggers a range of body changes which can eventually bring about a state of exhaustion. These can range from breathing becoming faster and shallower; you lose your appetite or food loses its taste; your skin can lose its colour or you can become flushed; your hands and feet can become cold. Also stress can make the immune system less efficient and one becomes susceptible to colds, flu and other infections. For all these responses to happen there are great demands on the nervous and endocrine system.

Unabated stress over a period of time can lead to more serious conditions. Some examples of stress-related disorders are gastritis, ulcerative colitis, irritable bowel syndrome, migraine, anxiety, depression, ulcers, hypertension, asthma, rheumatoid arthritis. The important thing is to recognize whether you are heading into, or are already in either of these patterns, to be proactive.

Reflexology can release tension and regulates breathing. The efficient functioning of the nervous and hormonal systems are vital in the maintenance of a healthy body. In a stress situation these systems become dysfunctional and there is discord in homeostatic harmony. Through the feet the nervous and endocrine systems are easily contacted, nurtured and harmonized once more. Reflex-ology can revitalize and rekindle your acuity. It can help you regain the ability to shift truthfully with the movement of life, to be receptive, accept reality, and accommodate what is going on in and around you. Reflexology can heighten your perception and state of awareness.

You can become more objective; a problem can be rationalised and everything falls into perspective.

As three quarters of dis-ease is created by stress of some sort, the state of relaxation and balance brought about by a sensitive reflexology treatment can have a profound effect on your general well-being. Remember that it is you having the treatment and it is you who allows the changes to take place which affect your current state.

Through Suzanne's work with SCOPE, she comes across people

with multiple sclerosis, motor neurone dis-ease, and some who are recovering from a stroke. Other people have spinal injuries, Parkinson's, Alzheimer's or cerebral palsy. Reflexology has been found beneficial by many people with such disabling conditions.

Reflexology does not aim to cure these conditions; it is not the 'magic bullet' people dream of. Yet take multiple sclerosis. Reflexology can play a big part in improving the quality of a person's life.

People with disabilities can feel anger about what has happened to them. From experience we have found that since reflexology works on more than one level, that is, it works on a mental, emotional and a physical level, many people have found that reflexology has helped them come to terms with disability.

The reflexologist is the catalyst, because people having reflexology do their own healing. As one person who had suffered a cerebral haemorrhage told Suzanne, 'I have now found a deep peace of mind which I have not experienced in years. Reflexology has also improved my memory. The left side of my body is stronger and functioning more effectively, and my walking has improved.' Another person with rheumatoid arthritis experienced more freedom of movement in the joints. He was also no longer constipated and felt more relaxed and very happy. He still had rheumatoid arthritis but his quality of life was better than it had been before reflexology.

A young man with cerebral palsy commented after treatment that he felt increased confidence as a person, better able to take charge of his life and felt more emotionally stable. His speech had become much clearer, the spasms in his legs decreased markedly and he was sleeping more deeply. His comment after the final treatment, as he then left the centre was that his whole frame of mind was relaxed. He was not the tense person he had been previously. However after some weeks without reflexology his body started stiffening up again, although his speech continued to improve and mentally he remained buoyant.

This shows that as people with chronic disablement may be on a maintenance medication for life, reflexology too needs to be ongoing for them. A man with rheumatoid arthritis found this to be true. 'When I had reflexology regularly I felt A1. Then when the treatment stopped for four months my general condition deterior-ated. Now I am back having the treatment once a week and again I feel A1.'

Reflexology has been found particularly valuable to people in wheelchairs. It is possible to have a treatment without having to transfer onto a couch, as required for other body work, although if one is able to transfer the treatment is more relaxing. Wheelchair users do not have the stimulus to reflex points in their feet experi-enced when weight-bearing. During walking the nervous, respirat-ory, blood and lymphatic systems of the body are stimu-lated as the feet make contact with the ground. With reflexology the body can be taken for a walk without going anywhere. For instance, as the hips and ankles reflect each other, gently rotating the ankles improves the energy flow through the hips and pelvic area where so much congestion can collect when sitting for long periods.

The important thing to remember when talking about disablement is that the person who has a particular condition is the specialist in how he or she feels and what his or her needs are. Questions to be addressed include are you getting enough sleep? What degree of pain or spasm are you coping with? Are you having breathing difficulties? What is your mobility factor? Are you incontinent? Are you just generally feeling low? If you are experiencing problems in these areas they are among the many situations which can respond to reflexology.

From the therapists point of view they may have had a good training, but have not had the opportunity to treat people with disabling conditions. But everyone needs to start somewhere and do not necessarily rule out a therapist who you feel drawn to because they have not had experience in treating your labelled condition. After all, they are not treating a condition but giving you a treatment. Your disablement is particular to you. Ideally you will be entering a partnership with your therapist, a partnership of discovery and learning for both of you. Reflexology gets people in touch with their bodies and brings about a heightened awareness, enabling the person to understand their condition better and live more comfortably by allowing changes to take place.

Reflexology can be useful used in conjunction with conventional medicine and conventional nursing practices in a hospital setting. Suzanne can clearly remember one woman she helped in a London hospital some years ago. This woman had had abdominal surgery and needed a second operation following complications. When she came out of theatre with an intravenous drip and a catheter from her bladder she was in a shocked state, and was not passing urine. Her fingers were swollen and she was indeed in some discomfort. Suzanne was not too sure what reflexology would achieve for this woman but offered her the chance of some. It is possible to release quite a lot of tension by working on the reflex area for the solar plexus. To counteract the shock, Suzanne worked on the area representing the adrenals, and then over the one for the pituitary

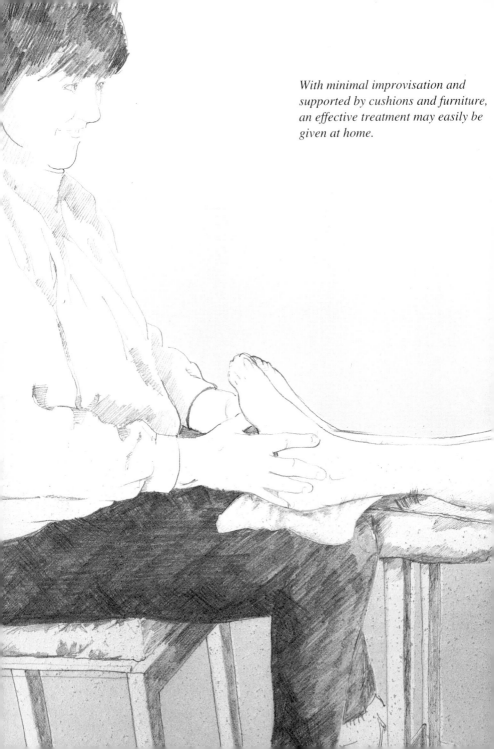

With minimal improvisation and supported by cushions and furniture, an effective treatment may easily be given at home.

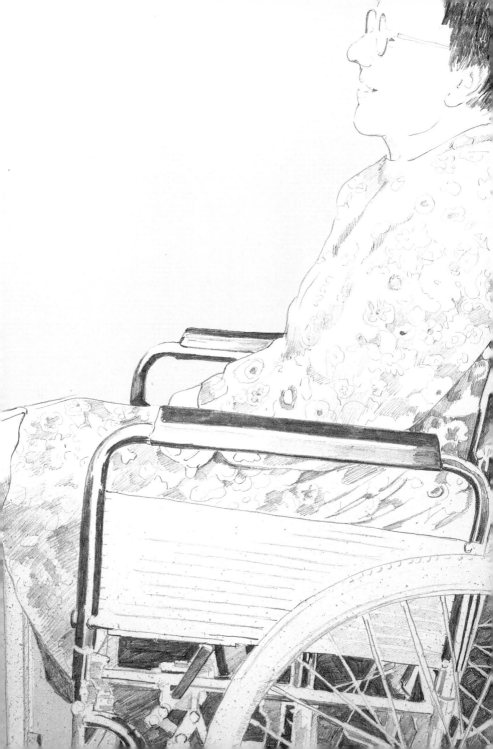

gland. Finally, she massaged the area for the kidney and bladder and could hear the urine draining away into the bag.

A simple form of reflexology has its place in the care of babies and young children, too. This is easy for parents to learn and use effectively for everyday problems when shown by a therapist.

Babies and children are very sensitive and respond to gentle stroking of the feet. They need a different type of touch from adults and respond well to calm, light touch. If you have had reflexology done on your feet it is not advisable to try to emulate that treatment with your child. You will be over-treating them and can cause discomfort. In addition, as babies respond to the parent's energy very quickly it is vital for the parent to be in a relaxed state before they start reflexology. While gently stroking the baby's feet the parent will feel even more relaxed and this peacefulness will be transferred to the child.

With a sick child you always consult your doctor first. But having said that reflexology can be helpful in relieving simple childhood problems, such as runny noses, and can be used in conjunction with medical treatment.

One baby had had a snuffly nose for two months almost since birth and when his mother had learned simple reflexology, she would gently massage his toes every time she changed his nappy. The toes relate to the nose, sinuses and breathing system in the head. In three days his breathing was quite free.

Reflexology can be used in caring for a disabled child. It can help family members accept the disablement and be active in assisting the child, as Florence Nightingale said, 'to use well every power that he or she has'. It can also allow a parent, carer or friend to take over the 'treatment' after a short period of tuition, after all, you are not treating an ill person, you are treating a person who happens to have a physical limitation.

One family, mother, father and older brother, found that by doing reflexology with the youngest member it helped them as a unit come to terms with disability. The mother explained that she and her husband were very frightened at first when they realised that their youngest son had cerebral palsy. 'It was as if we had never held a child or anything. We did not know how to pick him up and everyone was frightened to do anything with him. The reflexology helped us to come to terms with my son's disability. It gave me a lot of time just to sit there with him, very calmly. And it helped my son. He used to be miserable a lot at the beginning, very cranky. Now he's very placid and has less spasm, not nearly as stiff or tight. He just lies there and is quite relaxed about everything.'

As well as helping new lives to develop happily, the power of touch can be useful at the other end of the life cycle. It can enhance the quality of life for those who are ill, even with a terminal illness.

Being an accepted member of a group or family ensures security and stability that allows individual freedom, but with consideration for the family group as a whole. On many occasions illness is accompanied by a sense of loneliness and separation that increases the stress of being ill. A sensitive human being is well suited to assist a person who is concerned that he is separated from everyone else. We know of a family which was given strength and a feeling of involvement when members were taught how to give reflexology to their loved one who was dying of cancer. They were given peace as they travelled with him on the last journey together. The feeling of being nurtured and being able to nurture was strengthening for them all.

It is also essential that therapists do understand that there are times when reflexology is just too much for a sick person to bear. Enthusiastic therapists sometimes find this hard to understand. Some people simply cannot tolerate being touched when they are sick but are happy to have their feet massaged at other times. Therapists must be aware and sensitive enough to know when to treat and when to leave alone. It is an invasion of privacy and abusive to do reflexology with someone who does not want it.

Recently, Eilish's sister, the youngest in a family of three girls, was diagnosed as having advanced cancer. Eilish was there, and during those initial days following the news, helped her to make her will and plan for the future. One morning Eilish was distressed and very confused about how to proceed. So many concerned people around Margaret were trying to do something for her which only served to drain her energy.

Eilish asked herself what kind of person would her sister really need at this time when facing the possibility of imminent death. The answer was clear and brought Eilish great relief. She would like someone who was not distressed to be with her; someone who could just be there, attentive, listening and doing by not doing; someone who could help her adapt to the new situation and live accordingly.

Often a sick person is made more comfortable just by the presence of another. Of course, this means the presence of a person who is not preoccupied or distracted. Doing nothing in this frenetic world is often very difficult. Being present and available for someone is probably the greatest honour we can all give.

Therefore in some situations, simply by being there for a person, the reflexologist can aid the healing process. It is just another aspect of the reflexology partnership, the healing bond. The fact that someone is present purely in a listening capacity, not judging, not putting their own needs across, just allowing that person to gather their thoughts, can be so helpful. By doing that when the mood requires it, you are starting to build up a relationship of security and safety. If the person wants to speak they do so. If they do not, that is fine. In slowing down, a person can relax and in this way can identify and consider any anxiety or worries.

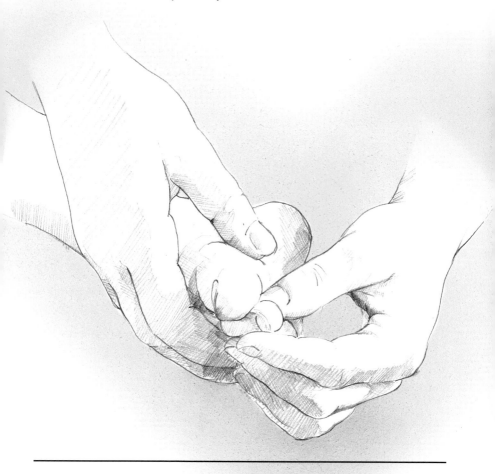

For us this type of partnership is the essence of this book. It is one that does not cause stress, offence, and at least, the minimum of discomfort for all concerned. When people are fortunate enough to be involved in such a partnership, we believe that reflexology can be of great benefit and value.

Over the past decade our understanding of reflexology has changed. Until recently most books gave a specific list of contra-indications when reflexology should not be carried out. The lists included infectious illnesses, high temperature, chronic and acute inflammation of the venous and lymphatic systems, unstable pregnancy, conditions that require surgery, heart conditions, diabetes and extensive fungal infections of the feet.

Yet we believe people experiencing such problems may well benefit from the gentle and comforting touch of a sympathetic therapist. They become more relaxed which in turn can help them consider any problems their particular medical condition has caused or will cause.

It used to be thought that you should not have reflexology soon after eating. It is all right to have a reflexology session after a meal and you don't need to wait until it is digested. In fact, reflexology brings relaxation and release that improves body function. The organs of digestion work more efficiently. You will feel energized by a session.

The stress-releasing effect of reflexology enhances the healing process, for example, both before and after surgery. Reflexology is always inappropriate when a person does not wish it. But there are other times when it may not be advisable because of a particular medical condition. In the case of someone having very fragile skin like in advanced diabetes or skin lesions in psoriasis when the skin is weeping, great care needs to be taken, and contact reflexology may not be desirable. This is when treating the hands can be considered. However, it is possible still to treat, without physical touch, through the energy field which we all radiate. This energy field, which has been scientifically proved by Kirlian photography, is being explored more fully as instruments become more sophisticated.

As a result, our knowledge of this previously mysterious world is growing. People who have had a limb removed often feel sensation in the toe that is not there. The energy imprint of the whole body remains intact even when a limb or organ is removed. 'Phantom limb pain' is a common manifestation of the reality of the energy imprint and not an illusion as previously thought. Effective reflexology treatments can be given in the energy field where the foot has been.

CHAPTER 5
HOW TO FIND YOUR THERAPIST

So while bearing in mind that the relationship between a therapist and a therapee is a partnership how do you find a therapist and begin to develop that healing bond?

The healing process starts even before treatment. The process began when you decided to try it. But it has to be your own decision. Do not succumb to another person's insistence that it would be good for you. It is also important initially to understand that ultimately it is not where any treatment is carried out, but how it is done. It can be a therapist's home or a practice in a clinic. What is vital is that you feel comfortable in a particular environment. You may prefer the 'cosiness' or intimacy of a therapist's home. You may prefer a therapist to visit your home if that is at all possible, or you may prefer a more formal relationship in a more clinical environment, in a room designed solely for the practice of complementary therapies.

As well as being comfortable with the environment you need to be at ease in the company of the therapist too. Change takes place when you are in a relaxed and trusting state.

Some people may well be anxious about finding a therapist. We feel that a personal recommendation is one of the best ways of starting to find the right therapist for your needs. You can also find a reflexologist by contacting organizations listed on page 94.

Some therapists also advertise in health food shops or health magazines. Even *Yellow Pages* covers reflexologists.

The Association of Reflexologists, for instance, publishes a referral register of practitioners for the benefit of members of the public wish to consult a qualified and experienced reflexologist. These members can be recognized by the letters M.A.R. or O.M.A.R. after their name. For those wishing to learn the art of reflexology, the association also publishes a list of recognized and accredited training schools. The therapists listed do not claim to cure, diagnose medical conditions or prescribe.

If you have a medical condition which is requiring constant medical monitoring and medication and are considering embarking on a course of reflexology it is advisable to discuss this with your G.P. as he or she is responsible for your healthcare. This is particularly important if you are a diabetic on insulin or being prescribed cortisone for any reason. In situations such as these, it is important that you inform your therapist. It is never wise to make changes in medication without discussing the strategy with your doctor; they will record any change of prescription.

Reflexologists do not treat specific ailments, but treat the person by stimulating and balancing the whole body. It is interesting that many people come to reflexology because of particular conditions, such as low back pain or tennis elbow, which may not have responded to other forms of treatment. They often find because of reflexology's balancing effects that during a course of treatment other more minor symptoms which they have just put up with resolve as well.

The reflexology partnership usually begins by a phone call. But something as simple and straightforward as that can put you on the right track. We are all intertwined. Or as one Indian writer put it, all things and beings in the universe are connected with each other, visibly or invisibly, and through vibrations a communication is established between them on all the planes of existence. Or more simply, we are all in the same soup together. Therefore to go to a therapist who is in a state of agitation cannot be advantageous. There can be shifts of energy between the therapist and you. If the therapist is in bad form that can drain your energy. A responsible reflexologist will not go ahead with an appointment if they themselves are not feeling well because it will affect the quality of the treatment. A treatment session is a two-way experience. Your relationship with the therapist and their relationship with you affects the outcome of the treatment. So that initial contact on the phone can be a useful introduction for both of you. Some therapists will answer the phone themselves while others have a receptionist or answering machine.

Your feelings and thoughts at this time are important information to help you find the therapist suited to you. How you react to their tone of voice, for instance, is important. If you do not feel reassured by the tone then there is a possibility that their whole therapy might have a similar effect on you. If the voice is rushed, official and impersonal, that may present you with a feeling of unease. Do you feel that the therapist is taking an interest in your call? If he or she is interested in you on the phone then the likelihood is that that same interest will be present during a reflexology treatment. These first impressions are lasting and set the tone of the relationship developed with the person seeking assistance.

Take into account some other aspects of your visit, too. If you are disabled it is vital that you ascertain if easy access is available. In some circumstances a home visit can be arranged.

How long is a treatment session likely to last? If you are going to be travelling by car, then it is worthwhile asking what the car parking arrangements are. You do not need the added worry if you have concerns about where you can park your car, for example, or whether the parking meter is going to run out.

You also need to discuss the area of payment as reflexology is not available generally on the NHS. If finance is difficult most therapists can agree to an effective compromise which is acceptable to both of you. This can be clarified during your first visit. Suzanne has been fortunate in having the opportunity to work for six years in a centre for people with disability, where clients could enjoy the experience and benefit of complementary therapies without having a financial burden to cope with. One wishes this to be the vision for the future. We have heard, however, of one Priority Care National Health Service Trust (a service supporting people with learning disability) which has recently developed a community reflexology service that is proving to be of value to the users and being respected by the medical profession. Perhaps this will herald a new approach to community care generally.

Each person coming for reflexology merits recognition that their needs, no matter how trivial they may seem, are important. At this stage there is no commitment on your part. If you feel uncomfortable, make a mental note and consider it later when making your choice.

This is more difficult in a large clinic as the receptionist presents their own personality and not that of the therapist. If you feel the need to make personal contact before embarking on a treatment session it should be possible to organize it.

The Meeting

Although no words are spoken the decor, seating, colours, texture, temperature, ventilation and lighting reflect the planning that went into the treatment area. What consideration has been given to your comfort? Is the place designed with the therapist in mind – or the therapee? It is conducive to the reflexology partnership if the reflexologist, no matter where the treatment is to be carried out, does accommodate your needs and has thought about them. It is helpful for you to be given privacy, or a private place, to prepare yourself. There should be a toilet nearby for you to use. You need to feel comfortable during the session. If you feel you want to wash your feet after a busy day, there will be facilities available to do that, but it is not a prerequisite to treatment.

Are there signs that the people coming here are really and genuinely wanted or is there a feeling that you are intruding? A lot of therapists work at home and some people are happy to go there. Others are happy to go to a formal clinic but the same basic considerations apply. This is not to be compared to a doctor's surgery or a hospital because the art of reflexology is based on a different way of alleviating distress. It is focused on touch which is done with the hands alone. As needles are not used nor the skin broken nor body cavities entered into, clinical aseptic conditions are not needed in the furnishings or clothing of therapists, nor is it necessary to wear gloves.

Having arrived for your first appointment, what are your impressions? Do you consider that you are being made to feel welcome and are you being put at ease? If you have no prior knowledge of reflexology you can expect a brief explanation of the therapy and how it works. This is a time when you can ask any questions you may have – there will also be other opportunities as the relationship develops. At this stage if you are feeling unsure about any aspect of treatment you can leave and the therapist will accept this.

The initial visit usually lasts about an hour and a half. Treatment itself can vary from any length up to an hour. You may be asked whether or not you want to tell the therapist why you have come. Do not feel you have to explain everything. You can say what you want to, or you can reveal nothing. The choice is yours. The therapee should feel free to tell the therapist anything about themselves that they wish in confidence.

Nevertheless some therapists feel that a detailed history of illness is important. They may want to know every illness you have ever had, any family medical problems such as people in your family who have had heart disease, diabetes and so on.

They may want to know about any surgery you have ever had. You may be asked about what you do for a living. You may be asked about your daily habits, such as the food you eat, how many cigarettes you smoke, how much alcohol you drink. Women may be asked about their menstrual cycle. But in reflexology we feel to emulate the medical model of history taking is not appropriate. Firstly because reflexologists are not usually medically qualified and also because our attitudes to treatment are quite different in any case.

A doctor's approach is to remove the symptom, while in reflexology the therapist does not focus on the symptom but the whole person with an innate ability to correct imbalances.

Symptoms are an indication that their equilibrium is disturbed. When this disturbance reaches a critical level medical intervention is essential to preserve life. We feel asking too many questions is an invasion of an individual's privacy.

The practice of medical record taking was introduced probably when people who had a nursing or medical background became involved with reflexology. As this re-emerging, but still very new, therapy grows it is evident that it is based on a different foundation from medical science, and efforts to make it fit into the medical model will dilute and destroy its potential to enhance our lives.

Deep inquiry could cause all manner of uncomfortable feelings. What does it feel like when the natural boundaries are being over-stepped? First there is the feeling of unease. This happens before there is any physical contact. The patient does not feel welcomed or made to feel that he or she is wanted for themselves. He or she feels invaded by some of the questions asked or inadequate because the patient feels he or she is not giving the right answers.

After this initial discussion, the actual treatment will commence. For some people taking off their shoes and socks, or shoes and tights can be a daunting thought. You may leave socks or tights on if you are not happy, or perhaps a little shy about letting someone else touch your bare feet. An effective reflexology treatment can be given with them on until you are comfortable enough to take them off. We do not believe that therapists need to wipe a person's feet before reflexology. Doing this can make a person feel their feet are unacceptable as they are. If you are doing people's feet and you are worried about hygiene and touching dirty feet, give it up and do something else.

Therapists usually wash their hands before giving a treatment which is in preparation and out of respect for the therapee. The state of a therapist's hands is indicative of their dedication to the therapy. Fingernails need to be short, hands warm and clean, and the skin in a good condition. Some therapists do have a problem with the temperature of their hands which can be corrected during their preparation. Sympathetic therapists will avoid anything distracting like jangling jewellery, or heavy perfume or aftershave, and their general appearance will be unremarkable.

Some reflexologists have background music playing as they feel it creates a mood of relaxation. Therapees can enjoy this but we feel it distracts your attention and separates you from what is going on between you and the therapist. Music is a therapy on its own. If you find your therapist has music playing and you find it distracting, request that it is stopped. The treatment offers you a chance to be attentive to what your body is telling you. Some therapists offer a footbath and that can be very relaxing before treatment.

Reflexology will be done while you are lying on a couch or in a reclining chair, with your body weight supported so that you can

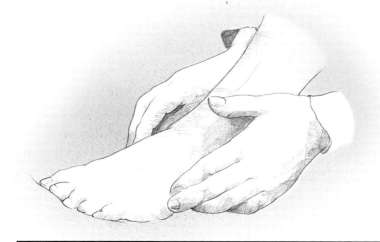

relax and your arms in a position you find comfortable. If by any chance lying or reclining is uncomfortable for you, then you can sit upright. A support under your knees eases tension at the base of your spine. Being comfortable helps you to get the most out of the treatment. So take notice if your belt or tie is fastened too tightly.

We feel seeing your own feet can be reassuring so that you can view what is going on if you want to and you will feel less vulnerable. But it is your choice; you can lie flat and look at the ceiling if you prefer.

You may be offered a blanket to put over yourself. Many people find this comforting and when in a state of relaxation you can lose body heat.

During treatment the reflexologist may use oil, powder, or cream that allows the hands to glide over the skin. Baby oil is not suitable as it does not allow the hands to move smoothly. Some reflexologists feel strongly against the use of creams or powder as they say it creates a barrier between you and them. We agree with their sentiments but believe that different approaches are necessary for different people.

Either way it is the intention and the nature of the touch that determines the treatment's effect. Some therapists do not allow their clients to talk during treatment. But in our experience this restriction can actually be stressful. They would argue that if you are talking about things which disturb you your body becomes tense and the treatment is not as effective. But you cannot exert such control over a person's mind. A therapee may not be communicating verbally what they are thinking, but they may still be thinking uncomfortable thoughts all the same.

Since some therapees will have no desire to talk, the choice

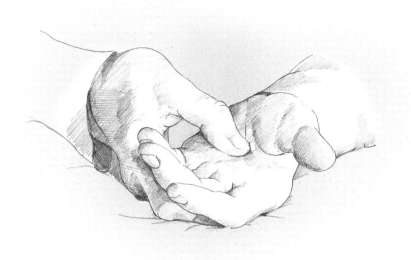

must be theirs. Others welcome the opportunity to have an attentive, neutral listener to share their one-sided conversation – their worries, fears, doubts, hopes, successes, moments of elation in trust and confidence. It can be such a freeing experience. And this release might never have come if they had not been allowed to speak.

Confidentiality is the basis of the reflexology partnership. When we confide in someone we are usually needing assistance with something which is troubling us. We are not able to come to a solution ourselves but voicing it to another person is often all that is necessary to clarify and resolve. The sum of the combined energy is more effective than trying to reach a resolution alone.

The actual reflexology treatment will be made up of a number of movements. There are various methods and systems but you should always feel safe and secure. Discomfort can occur in some areas of the feet and steps will be taken to alleviate it.

Usually at the beginning of a first session and before treatment really gets underway there are introductory movements to induce relaxation and to put the therapee at ease. This is an important preliminary procedure when the therapist and the new therapee can get to know each other while still maintaining a formal distance. The beginning of the session is an opportunity to allay any feelings of apprehension or uncertainty you might have felt about having your feet touched by a stranger.

It is also an opportunity to confirm your expectations that reflexology would be something you would enjoy and find worthwhile. Responses to these initial contacts set the tone for the type of massage used with you at this stage. Reflexology is about sensing rather than talking and deducing rationally. It is about care.

There are many ways a therapist can start treatment as it is such an individual therapy. Each therapist has his or her own way of working. There are times when the use of a lubricant is appropriate. There are many methods of how people use their fingers and the shape of the foot allows great variety, innovation and creativity. One of the classic movements is the caterpillar. This is a very precise movement which the therapist performs with the inner tip of the thumb. It is an effortless, creeping forward movement over the skin. It is almost like a regular, normal heartbeat, like breathing, and the movement will flow with the movement of the body. The effect of this action is to help restore and normalize body function.

Other movements include using all fingertips, the sides of the fingers, on-the-spot circular or stroking movements. You may experience some gentle loosening movements such as rotation of each individual toe, gentle stretching of the toes, rotation of the ankles, stretching of the ankle by moving it backwards and forwards. Pressing in and out of the ball of the foot with one hand while supporting it with the other is often a very soothing and comforting experience.

The reflexologist will usually ask you to let him or her know what you are feeling physically in your feet or how you feel inside. Do let them know how you feel as the treatment can be adapted accordingly. But do not feel concerned if you are unable to communicate in this way – this is a common experience.

Reflexologists have ways of trying to assess how you feel through your feet and bodily responses. If you are feeling uncomfortable about the session do say so.

On the other hand if there is any part of the treatment which you particularly enjoy or find beneficial and would like continued, do feel free to say that also.

The therapist is likely to ask you to let them know if anything he or she is doing is causing you discomfort. There will be times when you will experience discomfort, such as prickly sensations in your toes, or crunchy areas on the ball of the foot. As the therapist works over the areas the sensations will 'dissolve'. People often describe this as a good, relieving type of discomfort. They feel as if an energetic flow is released which creates a freedom. You may wonder how long you should carry on with reflexology. The answer is, it is up to you. You are the one who decides. You should discuss it with your therapist.

How often you should have a reflexology treatment varies from one individual to another and so many other factors are involved such as the accessibility of the therapist, transport, available time, finance etc., what your condition is at the time. In our experience starting with a treatment at least twice a week is a good idea although few people can manage that. Over time the intervals between each treatment can be extended to weekly then two weekly according to how you feel and what is possible. It is a very individual decision which needs to be made in relation to what is happening in the rest of your life.

Pressures from outside have a marked effect on our general well-being and changes in the frequency of treatments can be made to accommodate as necessary. In some situations it would be ideal to have a treatment daily for a period of time.

However, this can be difficult unless you have an in-house therapist. Some people function on bursts of regular treatment with gaps in between. If you are dependent on organizations like day centres or health authorities for the therapy it is not easy to have a say in treatment programmes, but it does no harm to voice one's needs as it may encourage more flexibility in the service if possible.

In our experience people who are dependent on continual drug treatment respond more slowly to the effect of reflexology. Some medications or physical conditions desensitize the feet; however, even though the client may not feel any or little sensation during the treatment, it does not mean that they are not benefiting by it. Sometimes it takes a number of treatments before a person's feet will register sensation and in some cases of paralysis, for example spinal injury, where sensation has been destroyed, that person will still benefit by reflexology.

When you feel more in touch with yourself you feel a greater harmony with the world. Everyday problems become less daunting and easier to resolve. It allows you to bring clarity of vision into your life. How this happens we are not sure of. There is some mystery attached – and what is wrong with having some mystery to life.

Many people are put off reflexology because it is a therapy of touch and because they do not like their own feet. They find them ugly, misshapen or are just not used to other people seeing them at close range. But feet are beautiful structures. You need to remember that your feet support your body weight. You cannot move any-where without them. And to expect them not to show any signs of wear and tear would be like an adult face with no lines on it. Hard skin is nothing to worry about either. Hard skin develops on the

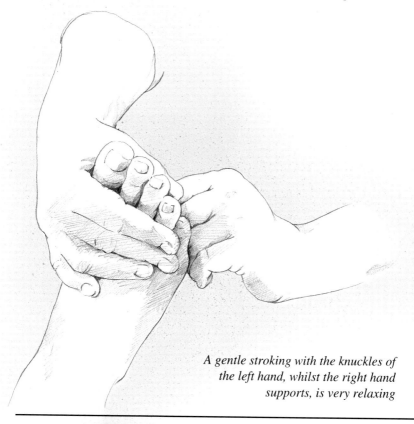

A gentle stroking with the knuckles of the left hand, whilst the right hand supports, is very relaxing

foot in the area reflecting the corresponding area of the body where the vital energy is not flowing freely. Hard skin is a natural protective mechanism. In the feet taking hard skin off does relieve the physical discomfort but it does not get to the root of the problem. During a course of treatment patches of hard skin can loosen and slowly peel away.

If you want to have a pedicure to remove it and then have reflexology that is fine. If that will make you feel more relaxed, it will be beneficial. But you do not have to.

Feet are nothing to be ashamed of. You can reduce any anxiety about your feet by taking a good look at them. We know that many of us never really look at their feet unless we want to check between the toes to see if the skin is healthy. By familiarizing yourself with your feet you will become less self-conscious of them and begin to fully appreciate and value them.

CHAPTER 6
HOW SIMPLE
REFLEXOLOGY CAN HELP
YOU HELP YOURSELF

You can practise reflexology on your own feet. Your relationship with your self is the foundation of your relationships with other people. So often we are too hard on ourselves by constantly pushing ourselves to do better or criticizing ourselves for not coping with life the way we think we should.

There are people who have daily gym workouts as a means to get fit. But some of these people seem to stand there chastizing themselves. We have watched them giving their own bodies a punishing workout – as if they feel their bodies have failed them.

Simple reflexology can be used to nurture yourself and support yourself in the true spirit of partnership. By giving yourself a reflexology treatment you are creating an opportunity to be kind to yourself and to cherish your own body.

We live more fully through other people than we do alone. So in many ways it is preferable to seek treatment from a reflexologist. There is energy exchange. You are being nurtured and are giving the other person a chance to expand their nurturing capabilities.

There are times to be with other people and there are times to be alone. Self-treatment is better than no treatment at all. It is a way of getting in touch with yourself. It is very valuable when used in conjunction with treatments as maintenance between sessions from a therapist. It feeds the process of change. You are taking a responsible, active role in the reflexology partnership.

Look at self-treatment as a way of unwinding. There are different ways of relaxing, reading a novel, going for a walk, listening to music – or doing your feet.

Through touch you can understand yourself better and things become clearer to you. It is not essential to know which reflex areas of your feet represent which areas of your body. You will intuitively know which areas of your feet will need more attention. You will feel areas of tenderness, of congestion, of hard skin and you will dwell slightly longer on these areas.

Self-treatment is a good exercise for the hands as they are moving and being used in physical activity which keeps them supple. Being able to help yourself, rather than always being helped, has a positive effect on your psyche. You are not helpless and you are able to help yourself.

How you treat yourself is how you should treat other people. It is a good idea first of all to massage your own hands and fingers, feeling them and observing their uniqueness. Have you have been appreciating them and giving them due care and attention?

Hands can be done anywhere, anytime, and when feet are inaccessible or a person is not able to bend to reach them. When you are driving and feeling tense you can stop somewhere safe and support one wrist with the other hand and rotate the supported hand. This relieves a lot of tension.

When massaging yourself hands are easier to do than the feet as you can sit with hands resting on your lap or supported on a table (with or without a cushion) in front, or lie comfortably with hands resting on your abdomen. Also there is no difficulty with intimacy when it is your own hands that you are touching. Many movements such as the 'finger walking', where there is forward progression, are easily adapted for self-treatment.

So many actions of touch are automatic. We do them without even thinking about it. Clasping our hands together with firm pressure, pressing fingertips together and pressing our temples with our fingers are all actions carried out with the intent of increasing our brain power!

Touch can be used to nurture ourselves but it can also be used to calm ourselves in specific situations. Just before a job interview is one such instance. You may be feeling so anxious and thinking of what you are going to say in an interview that it is probably the last thing you can imagine doing at this point. Nevertheless it is a remarkably effective calming technique.

Just find the place in the soft centre of your hand where you feel that the space goes on for ever and press in, relax out and pause. Do this cycle at the speed of relaxed breathing – which is about twenty times a minute.

The speed is much less than the rate of your own heartbeat which may be racing along at 80 to 90. The natural inclination is to move at that rate, so you will need consciously to concentrate on doing it more slowly. In doing so this will calm you, centre your attention and compose you.

This routine is also very effective when you cannot switch off and go to sleep. Start by doing the same in, out, pause sequence. Make sure your hand is in a relaxed position resting on your abdomen. You can do the cycle under the bedclothes so that you still keep warm and often it is not necessary to do both hands: by the time you have massaged one hand you will feel relaxed enough to fall asleep.

Massage is soothing and takes your mind off the fact that you are not sleeping. As well as pressing the centre of your palm you can use any rotating movements with your thumb to massage your hands. You can go all around the hand finger walking. You can massage your hands with your knuckles. At work you can use this relaxation technique. Your boss might be breathing down your neck all day. A boss might use it to relieve the stress of management.

There are many times when we can massage our own feet. As a regular part of caring and attending to our feet. Following a long, arduous walk, a long period of standing, a stressful situation where you felt unsupported and unfairly criticized, for example during a row with your partner or a relative. Other beneficial times include after sports, when your feet have been in shoes for a long time, sitting without moving, at the end of a tiring day, any long journey, following a journey – especially for the driver who has been driving on a motorway and has had a buildup of tension in the muscles of neck and shoulders.

Cherishing ourselves can be done any time. Spending some time massaging our own feet when we feel great is a wonderful way of maintaining this state of well-being.

Quite a lot of people do not like their feet, or are shy about them and self-massage and care is an easy way of exploring them, accepting and becoming friendly with them. While you are contacting them, touching and feeling them, consider how they serve you, notice their structure and how wonderfully made they are.

An article in *The Times* highlighted that a survey done in 1991 showed that the average person takes 18,000 steps a day, and walks 70,000 miles in a lifetime. Bearing this in mind it is easy to see why our feet need regular attention but we usually do not give them attention until they let us down. Any extra care we give them in addition to washing and cutting our toenails is beneficial. When this is done fairly regularly people become more in tune with their feet, notice changes and respond compassionately when there is stiffness or aching.

Over a period of time, as a person becomes more familiar with their feet he or she observes changes in the texture or colour of the skin, temperature or mobility of the foot. When that person reflects there are usually signs of changing patterns in his or her way of living.

There is a better understanding of ourselves, an enhancement of our relationships and a more spontaneous communication with other people.

Through self-treatment we become more aware of our feet and at the same time of our bodies. We can respond to signals such as tiredness. We rest, and then we are restored.

Of course, none of this is instead of seeking medical attention should one feel it is necessary and symptoms persist.

To massage your feet you need ideally to find some time when you are not going to be interrupted. Reflexology with a therapist after a meal is OK but when it comes to self-treatment it is preferable, and more comfortable, if you have not just had a large meal because of the position you may need to adopt. Even ten minutes is valuable and can make all the difference between tearing your hair out and acting calmly. Giving your full attention to what you are doing is a benefit that renews us.

In certain situations such as a crisis or pain it can be used as a 'first aid'. Toothache responds well when pressure is applied to the corresponding place in the toes. It is easy to find the area in the toe which relates to the tooth, as it is usually quite painful, and is helpful until a visit to the dentist for expert advice and treatment.

For some people self-treatment is a good way of relaxing. When we are relaxed the body produces endorphins which can crudely be called 'natural painkillers'. Endorphins are stored and called into action when needed. They cannot be made when a state of alert is on so it is vital that they are regularly topped up to ensure they are plentiful should a crisis occur. When the crisis is over they can then be replenished as soon as possible and kept in storage until they are required. Relaxation in this way can be used as a 'first aid' measure.

Start with a bath, shower or foot bath if you wish. When you are ready to massage your feet you need to sit comfortably with your back well supported.

You can massage the top of your foot or you can massage the sole in turn. If you wish to do this then place a pillow under your knee for support while you turn your foot upwards so that the top of the foot is resting on your thigh and the sole of your foot is in front of you.

You can use any plain base oil – grapeseed or almond are good examples. Oil helps you move your hands more smoothly over the skin. You want to use an oil that allows freedom of movement which is why olive oil is perhaps too viscous and baby oil is not lubricant enough. Try not to interrupt contact with your foot and try to keep your movements fluid.

It is easy to forget how three-dimensional the foot is. You will

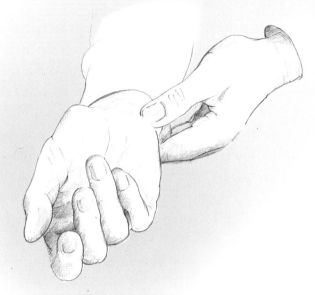

find it pleasant to massage the top of your feet and, although it is not considered to be related to the rest of the body in the same way as the sole, the massage still permeates through to the organs on the sole.

Support the foot with one hand. Gently move your toes with one hand and feel what is happening to them. The more you relax the more your toes will be able to move. Support the ankle by holding your hand over it and gently rotate your foot by holding the toes and the ball of the foot. Massage around the heel area, under the foot, endeavour to cover the whole foot.

You can use all your fingers. You can use either side edge of your fingers. This is more relaxing than using the fingers straight on. You can stroke down the sole of your foot with your knuckles or a soft fist. These are lovely things to do. Press your thumbs against the ball of your foot. Support your foot with your thumbs and walk the fingers over the top of the foot.

Endeavour to proceed in a forward direction. Working backwards creates a dragging effect – all fluid action is lost.

You can just hold your foot. You can support it. Cup it in your hands. Comfort it. Go gently in between the toes and over the ball of the foot which will help relax tension in your neck and shoulders. Feel underneath your toes. If you just give each toe a massage you are working the zones of your body. Work your way along the whole bony ridge on the inside of your foot which is like massaging your spine.

Flex your foot up and down. Rotating your ankle releases energy in the pelvic area. But do not force it. Go as far as that ankle is allowing you to go. Do not think I am going to force this ankle to move. Do not keep at it.

Try to cover the whole foot with rhythmic movements so that your whole body feels attended to. Sit with your hand covering the bottom of your foot. It is a fascinating thing because you can feel a movement of energy and warmth radiating throughout your body. Giving yourself individual attention in this way brings you in touch with your whole self. There are so many different techniques. Yet it is not the technique but the intent. It is not what you do but how you do it that matters.

A lot of people only acknowledge their feet as the two things at the end of their legs. They only become aware of their importance when something goes wrong. That is a little late. If you care for your feet now they will serve you well.

When you do massage your own feet, you will be interested to experience the different sensations you can feel. You will find that changes do take place. You may feel sensations of pins and needles, numbness, tingling, you may feel little crystals under the skin.

Some areas of the foot may feel warmer than others. You may feel tightness and stiffness. Sometimes an area of skin looks red, or shiny and taut, as if it could be damaged if treated roughly. Take care.

Do not push hard against an area that is sore. Your body is telling you to be gentle with it. On repeated treatments changes appear. Areas that had been sensitive are now less so. There can be changes in colour, temperature and texture. Hard skin can peel away.

There are times when as well as treating yourself you can treat others even if you are not professionally trained. As we are all endowed with the sense of touch there are many times when it is invaluable. Often it is the 'untrained' who intuitively are sensitive to the needs of others and can sense the areas in the feet which need attention. There is no reason to hold back when we feel touch is the right thing to do in a given situation because we are not trained.

When we watch television together, for example, why not take this moment of shared relaxation to relax even more. This is a good time for just holding each other's feet if we feel tired. After a day at work people in the family can 'do' each others feet and or hands in the evening.

Someone who knows nothing about the art of reflexology can be very helpful by simply responding to help another human being if the person is in distress. Do not hold back because you think you know nothing. You do not have to have knowledge to be able to comfort another person. The touch of a warm hand is calming and comforting and is therapeutic. It is how we are made.

CONCLUSION

Reflexology is a simple, safe, non-invasive therapy. No tools or implements are required. A pair of sensitive, willing hands and a willing recipient are all that are needed. There is a growing demand for this therapy with its approach allowing time for two people to communicate through touch, where words are often unable to convey what has happened or is happening.

The reflexology partnership is a non-verbal communication between two people which supports and validates the exchange of energy between them. This type of partnership is part of an exciting journey. It is a journey of discovery and of a heightened awareness of yourself rather than a journey that is mapped out to effect dramatic change.

The reflexology partnership aims to bring you in total harmony, in complete balance and at one with yourself. Just think of the horse, the rider and the reins. They form a unit in harmony and partnership which functions only as a whole.

For us the relationship between therapist and therapee works in the same way. Reflexology is a matter of the moment, responding to the needs of a person as shown in the feet. It should not be a matter of a therapist wanting to heal in order to satisfy his or her own altruistic need.

Some years ago one man with Aids told Eilish that he felt very uncomfortable when at a meeting strangers kept coming up to him and hugging him. He felt it was an invasion of his privacy and he was unable to say that he did not want to be hugged. Those doing the hugging were so carried away with their own needs they were insensitive to how distressed the recipients of these patronizing actions felt.

This is a good example of people being blinded by their own need and harming in the process. In the reflexology partnership, the only needs that should be evident are the needs of the person wanting reflexology. Our vision of such a partnership is about a therapist having the ability to read what the feet are saying about a person's needs and responding to those needs. Each individual situation and session is unique.

A therapist goes into a session without any expectations and empty of his or her own needs. If the therapist is looking for results there is happiness on his or her part when there is improvement and distress when there is deterioration. Wanting to create results is unhealthy. Wanting to change another person to make them be as you wish is selfish. It creates a division or separation between therapist and therapee, hindering spontaneous communication.

Spontaneous communication through touch brings with it many benefits. It can bring relief for many people without administering foreign substances into the body. Feet are easily accessible and the effects of a reflexology treatment can be felt throughout the body, including the mental and spiritual levels. We believe that reflexology, as a therapy, has a place on its own. But it can go hand in hand with orthodox medicine and can enhance its role in enriching the quality of life.

In reflexology change can be subtle and the body can move with and accommodate these changes without consciously registering what is going on. It can be that these changes have to be pointed out by someone else. 'I was watching you walk down the street and you had a spring in your step I had not noticed before.'

USEFUL ADDRESSES

The Association of Reflexologists
27 Old Gloucester Street
London WC1 3XX

British Reflexology Association
Monks Orchard
Whitbourne
Hereford and Worcester WR6 5RB
Telephone: 01886 821207
Send cheque or postal order for £1.50 for a register of qualified members

British Register of Complementary Practitioners
P.O. Box 194
London SE16 1QZ

British School of Reflex Zone Therapy
87 Oakington Ave
Wembley Park
London HA9 8HY
Telephone: 0181 908 2201
Send SAE for register of qualified practitioners

The British School of Reflexology
The Holistic Healing Centre
92 Sheering Road
Old Harlow
Essex CM17 0JW
Telephone: 01279 429060

Reflexologists Society
127 Bullbrook Drive
Bracknell
Berkshire RG12 2QR

The Scottish School of Reflexology
2 Wheatfield Road
Ayr, KA7 2XB
Telephone: 01292 287142